Managir
and

M000208339

This revised edition of *Managing Hot Flushes and Night Sweats* offers up-to-date and evidence-based information about the menopause and about hot flushes and night sweats, which are the main reason that women seek medical help.

The four-week self-help guide uses cognitive behavioural therapy, providing information and strategies for managing hot flushes and night sweats, as well as stress and sleep. The guide is interactive with exercises and homework tailored to women's individual circumstances and lifestyles. It challenges myths about menopause and aging and provides better understanding of flushes which in turn reduces stress and improves post-menopausal well-being. The various chapters discuss processes of identification and modification of triggers of hot flushes and offers tips to women on dealing with hot flushes in social and work situations.

The guide can be as effective as eight hours of group CBT and will help women who want to try a non-medical treatment that is brief and effective without side effects, or just want to be better informed.

Myra Hunter is emeritus professor of clinical health psychology at the Institute of Psychiatry, Psychology and Neuroscience, King's College London. She has worked with women in a clinical and research capacity for over 35 years, and her research on menopause has established her as an international expert in the field.

Melanie Smith is a highly specialist clinical psychologist working within a physical health context. She was lead therapist on MENOS 1&2 CBT trials for well women and women experiencing hot flushes and night sweats following breast cancer treatment. Melanie works at the Manchester and Salford Pain Centre and provides CBT training to health professionals working with women with menopause symptoms.

Managing Hot Flushes and Night Sweats

A Cognitive Behavioural Self-help Guide to the Menopause

Second Edition

Myra Hunter and Melanie Smith

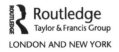
Routledge
Taylor & Francis Group

LONDON AND NEW YORK

Second edition published 2021
by Routledge
2 Park Square, Milton Park, Abingdon, Oxon OX14 4RN

and by Routledge
52 Vanderbilt Avenue, New York, NY 10017

Routledge is an imprint of the Taylor & Francis Group, an informa business

© 2021 Myra Hunter and Melanie Smith

The right of Myra Hunter and Melanie Smith to be identified as authors of this work
has been asserted by them in accordance with sections 77 and 78 of the Copyright,
Designs and Patents Act 1988.

First edition published by Routledge 2014

British Library Cataloguing-in-Publication Data
A catalogue record for this book is available from the British Library

Library of Congress Cataloging-in-Publication Data
Names: Hunter, Myra, author. | Smith, Melanie, 1975– author.
Title: Managing hot flushes and night sweats : a cognitive behavioural
    self-help guide to the menopause / Myra Hunter and Melanie Smith.
Description: Second edition. | Milton Park, Abingdon, Oxon ; New York,
    NY : Routledge, 2021. | Includes bibliographical references and index.
Identifiers: LCCN 2020014077 (print) | LCCN 2020014078 (ebook) | ISBN
    9780367430252 (hardback) | ISBN 9780367853037 (paperback) | ISBN
    9781003000761 (ebook)
Subjects: LCSH: Menopause—Popular works. | Cognitive therapy—Popular
    works. | Self-care, Health—Popular works.
Classification: LCC RG186 .H7837 2021 (print) | LCC RG186 (ebook) |
    DDC 618.1/75—dc23
LC record available at https://lccn.loc.gov/2020014077
LC ebook record available at https://lccn.loc.gov/2020014078

ISBN: 978-0-367-43025-2 (hbk)
ISBN: 978-0-367-85303-7 (pbk)
ISBN: 978-1-003-00076-1 (ebk)

Typeset in New Century Schoolbook
by Apex CoVantage, LLC

Visit the eResources: www.routledge.com/9780367853037

Dedication

In memory of Mary Gwyn Hunter
(30.11.1921 to 24.12.2012)

and

To Mum – Jane Smith – for your strength and dedication

Contents

Foreword

The process underpinning the menopause is a normal phase in women's lives but like others it is also one that can present some challenges. This book enables women to learn from the huge leaps forward in knowledge from psychological research. In particular it focuses on how our thinking affects our responses to menopausal changes. It constitutes a radical new way of viewing the menopause and managing any impact.

Making sense of any phenomenon, particularly something that is a highly personal experience, is the key to successful adjustment to change. Professor Hunter and Dr Smith provide a truly accessible and informative account of current knowledge relating to the menopause and its implications. It's not all about hormones. There is the history and the beliefs from different societies and how these can affect experience. But it is the focus on the published evidence that is the real key to the quality of this book. We are presented with the important developments in scientific understandings all simply explained. The myths of universal negativity are challenged, but there is constant recognition of and support for the individual differences in experiences.

The self-help programme is fully grounded in Professor Hunter's extensive and impressive published work on the topic. Essentially the programme is eminently doable. The reader is guided through the different elements that contribute to distress. At every point the exercises are fully explained and there are illustrations with quotes from women from a range of different circumstances. Every woman will find something that relates to her own experience. One of the most beneficial elements can be just understanding that one is not alone, that these are shared experiences and even more importantly that yes, there are ways of 'managing the menopause' that can be learned. This is something that anyone can do so long as they ensure they allocate the time and recognise that these are skills which do not develop overnight but require some effort and perseverance. The benefits of developing these skills are not just for the menopause. They are solidly grounded in cognitive behavioural psychology, which describes the fundamental links between bodily responses, thoughts, feelings and behaviours. These are understandings that can be of life-long help and improve well-being in all sorts of stressful circumstances.

This book is written by women for women, but partners and children are also important as they can both influence women's experiences by their own expectations and responses to the menopause. This should also be required reading for family members so that they can understand what the menopause really is and support women in the changes they are making.

Finally, maybe we need as a society to reconsider how we view the menopause and see this as just a normal, manageable and positive change in life and indeed the door to a menstrual cycle–free phase of life. We also need to value the older woman, her experience and wisdom.

Please read on, as your menopausal experiences will certainly seem different on your completion of this book.

Pauline Slade, Professor in Clinical Psychology and Consultant Clinical Psychologist University of Liverpool

Acknowledgements

We would like to thank all the women who have taken part in our research studies over the years and especially those who participated in our recent trials and provided such detailed and useful feedback. We are grateful to colleagues who contributed to the research over the past 30 years, including Lih-Mei Liao, Shirley Coventry, Beverley Ayers, Eleanor Mann, Janet Balabanovic, Evi Stefanopoulou, Joseph Chilcot, Sam Norton, Deborah Fenlon and Claire Hardy. Thank you also to Daradi Patar and Joanne Forshaw at Routledge for their helpful support and advice.

Grateful acknowledgement is made to the following for permission to include previously published material:

Figure 2.1 and Figure 4.1 'The thermoneutral zone (TNZ) and hot flushes' have been adapted and reproduced from Archer *et al.* (2011), Climacteric, with kind permission of Informa Healthcare.

Figure 4.2 and Figure 5.1 'A cognitive behavioural model of hot flushes' have been adapted and reproduced from Hunter (2003), *Journal of Reproductive and Infant Psychology*, with kind permission of Taylor and Francis.

Figure 6.1 'Stages of sleep' has been reproduced from LucidDreamExplorers (http://ygraph.com/chart/2076). Permission to use the chart is granted by Bulb Media on the condition that it is linked back to: www.LucidDreamExplorers.com/dreamscience/.

Excerpts from Hunter and O'Dea (1997) Menopause: Bodily changes and multiple meanings, in Ussher (ed.) *Body Talk: The Material and Discursive Regulation of Sexuality, Madness and Reproduction*. London: Routledge, pp. 199–222, reprinted with kind permission of Taylor and Francis Books (UK).

Note

Throughout the book any names of women have been changed for the sake of anonymity.

Introduction

If you have bought this book, you are likely to be having hot flushes and/or night sweats, and the first thing to bear in mind is that you are not alone. It is estimated that around 47 million women go through menopause each year worldwide (Hill 1996) and that 70–80 per cent of women in the UK and the US experience hot flushes and night sweats during the menopause (Hunter and Rendall 2007). Of these, over half will seek some kind of medical or non-medical help. Although we are talking a lot about 'symptoms', we view the menopause as a normal part of a woman's life rather than a medical problem. However, we appreciate that many women struggle to deal with frequent, intense hot flushes and night sweats and the impact that they can have on sleep, mood and daily life. Just as childbirth is a natural part of women's lives, there is a range of experience, and women should not feel like 'failures' if they do not sail through it or if they need some help to deal with it.

This new edition of our book provides an up-to-date guide to managing menopausal symptoms that can impact on quality of life, especially at work where women often find that they are more challenging to deal with (Griffiths and Hunter 2015). This self-help guide is for women who are seeking a non-medical treatment, or an alternative to hormone replacement therapy (HRT), for troublesome hot flushes and night sweats. It is also written for women who are experiencing these symptoms following breast or gynaecological cancer treatment, for working women, for women who are going through an early menopause and also for health professionals working with women who have menopausal symptoms. The book is based on cognitive behavioural therapy (CBT), which provides information and practical ways to change beliefs and attitudes and to develop helpful ways to deal with hot flushes and night sweats. We hope that it will be useful if you are having problematic symptoms but also if you just want to be better informed.

For some years, HRT has been the main medical treatment offered to women seeking help for hot flushes during the menopause. However, uptake of HRT almost halved following the publication of clinical trials of hormone treatments in 2002 and 2003 (Menon *et al.* 2007) – particularly the Women's Health Initiative (WHI) (Rossouw *et al.* 2002), which suggested that HRT is associated with a small but increased risk of breast cancer and strokes (www.nhlbi.nih.gov/whi/). Since then there have been heated debates about the methods and the findings of these studies in scientific journals and in the media. The first NICE (National Institutes of Health and Care Excellence) guidance on menopause for UK health professionals and women was published in 2015. The guidance states that for women under 60 years old who have symptoms, the risks of HRT are relatively small and usually outweighed by the benefits (www. nice.org.uk/guidance/NG23). A central theme of the guidance is the need to inform women of the risks and benefits of HRT so that they can make appropriate treatment choices. NICE also advises that women should be offered information about both medical and non-medical treatments.

While many non-hormonal treatments are available, the claims made for some have not been supported by strong evidence, and others have side effects (NICE 2015b). We believe that women should have up-to-date information about the treatments available to them so that they can make their own choices about treatments.

With colleagues, Myra Hunter has conducted clinical research developing non-medical treatments for women going through the menopause for many years. In the mid-1980s she spent several years working as a clinical psychologist with doctors at one of the first menopause clinics in the UK, at King's College Hospital in London. At that time there was little research on this topic, so her PhD focused on the experience of women during the menopause transition, and she has continued this work for over 35 years. In the 1990s, together with colleagues, she developed a non-medical treatment for menopausal hot flushes, based on CBT (see Chapter 3), and over time this treatment has been improved and tested in clinical trials.

She has developed group and self-help forms of CBT for menopausal symptoms and tested these treatments in clinical trials between 2008 and 2018 with over 1,000 women. Melanie

Smith carried out the CBT for hot flushes in these studies. The results show that the treatment is effective for women experiencing hot flushes during the menopause, for working women and also for women who have hot flushes following breast cancer treatments (Hunter and Liao 1996; Ayers *et al*. 2012; Mann *et al*. 2012; Duijts *et al*. 2012 Hardy *et al*. 2018a; Atema *et al*. 2019). We found that this self-help CBT guide was as effective as the group CBT and that both reduce the impact of hot flushes and night sweats with additional benefits to quality of life. Based on this work, CBT for menopausal symptoms has been recommended in a Position Statement by the North American Menopause Society (NAMS 2015), and by NICE (2015b) for anxiety and depressed mood during the menopause.

Because women often seek help during menopause when they are feeling overwhelmed by a combination of hot flushes and night sweats, sleep problems and stress, this book targets stress, hot flushes, night sweats and sleep problems using CBT. The book is divided into two main sections:

1 information about menopause, hot flushes and CBT; and
2 the CBT self-help guide.

We hope that, by offering evidence-based and balanced information and strategies to manage these common symptoms, the book will be both helpful and empowering. Women who have used the CBT self-help guide describe feeling more confident about dealing with the menopause and, in some cases, about their lives in general. The scope of the book does not include giving medical advice, such as the pros and cons of medical treatments; it is best to discuss this with your doctor because advice will be different for individual women.

Chapters 1 and 2 provide information about the menopause and hot flushes and night sweats, while Chapter 3 describes the cognitive behavioural approach. These introductory chapters explain the biological and the psycho-social changes that occur during the menopause transition, i.e. a bio-psycho-social approach. We describe cultural differences in experience of the menopause and psychological and social influences on menopausal symptoms. We also aim to challenge myths about menopause and ageing, and to provide information and advice about common concerns during the menopause, including sexual function, weight gain, memory and osteoporosis.

Women's experiences of menopause vary enormously, and while some women have no hot flushes at all, others do have debilitating symptoms that affect sleep and the quality of their lives in general. In the same way that women approaching childbirth find it helpful to be prepared, women approaching and going through the menopause can benefit from evidence-based information and advice too. But compared with childbirth, the menopause is still difficult to talk about in public, and women describe feeling embarrassed and fear negative reactions from others. Despite calls from women to challenge the 'menopause taboo', there is a long way to go – menopause is associated with quite negative meanings still. This is particularly true for women in social situations and at work – where many women feel that they have to hide symptoms for fear of ridicule and stigma.

Even in the twenty-first century, the menopause can still be difficult to discuss, and information is often polarized – we commonly see in the media extreme examples of women either embracing the menopause positively or having a whole host of problems requiring medical treatment. The impact of social media has been positive in providing women with means to talk more openly about menopause and network with other women, but again information can be diverse, conflicting and confusing. By including quotes from the women who participated in our research, we hope that the book will provide a range of real-life perspectives and help you to see that others are in the same boat and dealing with similar issues.

Before presenting the self-help guide, there will be a brief overview of CBT outlining some basic cognitive behavioural principles and providing answers to frequently asked questions regarding the use of psychological interventions or self-management approaches for physical health problems.

The main part of the book is the self-help guide for managing hot flushes and night sweats, which is completed over four weekly sessions. This section very much 'stands alone', so if you are well informed already or impatient to move on to the treatment, you can go straight to this section. The information in the self-help guide also summarizes some of the information that is provided in earlier chapters so that you have all the relevant details just where you need them. However, either way, it is best to work through the guide methodically once you have started the four-week programme.

The guide is interactive with a focus on building strategies tailored to your specific circumstances through active cognitive and behavioural change. You can develop your own individualized self-management plan by learning about the physiological mechanisms of hot flushes, the role of stress and stress management strategies, cognitive behavioural strategies to manage hot flushes and strategies to improve sleep and night sweats. The guide finishes with a review and a maintenance plan focused on relapse prevention, i.e. ways to help you maintain the positive changes you have made. At the end of each chapter (Weeks 1 to 4), you are invited to assign yourself weekly 'homework' in order to practise and consolidate CBT skills prior to the next session. You will be encouraged to practise relaxation and paced breathing to manage hot flushes and night sweats by using the audio link provided. A final section includes links to useful resources.

1

The menopause
A bio-psycho-social transition

What is the menopause?

The menopause occurs on average between the ages of 50 and 51 in most Western cultures, and literally refers to a woman's last menstrual period. The term originally comes from the Greek words 'menos' and 'pausos', which mean 'month' and an 'ending'. In this case, the 'ending' refers to the cessation of ovulation – the production of fertile eggs or ovum – and therefore fertility, and it also marks a change in life stage for many women. Most women will go through the menopause, although for some the timing of the menopause is influenced by surgery or disease. Hot flushes and night sweats (the medical term for these is 'vasomotor symptoms') are the other main physical signs of menopause.

The last menstrual period takes place within a gradual process of biological change, occurring at the same time as other age-related changes and within varied social and cultural contexts. Consequently, the menopause happens at several levels – the biological, psychological, social and cultural (Hunter and Rendall 2007). Perhaps because it typically occurs at the age of 50, during midlife, when most women are working, and life demands and stresses typically accumulate, the menopause has been associated with role and social changes for women. However, this is not necessarily the case for everyone. As we will see in the following sections, what is happening in a woman's life is very varied and can influence how she feels about approaching the menopause. Increasingly, the role of personal and lifestyle factors is being acknowledged and understood when considering how women experience the menopause. There is a gradual shift away from a primarily biomedical approach to the consideration of the influence of the psycho-social and cultural factors in women's lives that can shape the menopause transition (Judd *et al.* 2012) (see Figure 1.1).

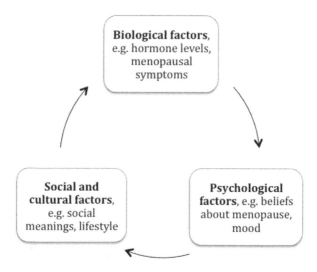

Figure 1.1 A bio-psycho-social model of factors influencing experience of the menopause

For example, for one woman the menopause meant that she no longer had to deal with having heavy periods, and this was a relief to her; for her friend, however, whose night sweats had woken her every night and disturbed her sleep for several months, the menopause felt like an ordeal. Similarly, for a woman who is planning to have children in her 40s, an early menopause is likely to have a major impact, whereas for a woman who has already had her family, the issue of fertility may be less relevant. However, for many women, uncertainty and some anxiety about what is happening or is likely to happen to them is a real concern, and the impact of accumulation of stresses during midlife should not be underestimated.

Some definitions

Menopause is defined by doctors and researchers as the permanent ending of menstruation and is said to have occurred when a woman has not had a menstrual period for one year. While the hormonal changes that accompany menopause happen over a number of years, the stages of the menopause transition are generally based on patterns of menstrual periods:

- Premenopause is defined by regular menstruation.
- Perimenopause includes the phase immediately before the menopause and the first year after menopause and is

defined by changes in the regularity of menstruation during the previous 12 months.

- Postmenopausal women are those who have not menstruated during the previous 12 months.

It can be difficult to fit all women easily into this classification; for example, if you have had a hysterectomy (removal of the womb), had surgery to remove your ovaries or are taking hormone therapy, you will not be having natural menstrual periods. Women in these categories tend to be classified separately because, for them, menstruation would not be a reliable indicator of menopause.

In 2012, the Stages of Reproductive Aging Workshop (STRAW) created a better system to describe stages of reproductive ageing across the whole life cycle (Harlow *et al.* 2012). It is based on evidence and reflects the parallel changes in menstruation, hormonal changes and experience of hot flushes and night sweats across women's lifespans.

The term 'perimenopause' is commonly used to refer to the menopause transition and early postmenopause, since this is the stage during which most physical changes occur. The STRAW definitions have also increased our understanding of when menopause occurs and how long it typically lasts (see Box 1.1).

Box 1.1 Stages of Reproductive Aging (STRAW) definitions

- **Reproductive stage**: includes menarche (onset of menstrual periods) with variable menstruation initially; it can take several years for regular menstrual cycles to develop, and these are usually every 21 to 35 days. Across this phase – typically from adolescence to late 40s – fairly regular menstruation continues, but there can be some changes in flow (sometimes becoming heavy) and in the length of the cycle.
- **Menopause transition**: includes early transition (regular menstruation but changes in menstrual cycle length) as well as late menopause transition (two or more missed menstrual periods and at least one interval of 60 days or more between menstrual periods), which happens one to three years before the final menstrual period. During this stage follicle-stimulating

hormone (FSH) levels tend to rise (this hormone is working hard to try to produce ovulation) and oestrogen levels start to reduce. Hot flushes are likely to occur during the late menopause transition.

• **Menopause**: the last menstrual period (LMP).
• **Postmenopause**: this stage is divided into early (up to six years after the LMP) and late (the subsequent years). Early postmenopause is characterized by hormonal changes and hot flushes, which tend to stabilize during the late postmenopause.

Additional terms – such as 'climacteric syndrome' and 'menopause syndrome' – have been used, mainly by doctors, to refer to a range of physical and emotional experiences that may or may not be related to hormone or menstrual changes. These include hot flushes, vaginal dryness, loss of libido, depression, anxiety, irritability, poor memory, loss of concentration, mood swings, insomnia, tiredness, aching limbs, loss of energy and dry skin. These will be discussed in later sections but – apart from hot flushes, night sweats and vaginal dryness – the other symptoms are not necessarily a result of menopause and, if they occur, may well have other causes as well, such as stress, ageing and lifestyle.

'The change' or 'change of life' is a commonly used term in Western cultures, reflecting the view that the meaning of the menopause is closely associated with general psychological and social adaptations women experience at midlife. 'Midlife crisis' also suggests that this stage might coincide with dramatic changes in personal and social relationships and with life events such as illness, caring for (and the death of) parents, dealing with adolescents and children leaving home, as well as reaching the age of 50. We tend to view menopause as a period of transition with pros and cons, just like other life transitions for women, such as adolescence and childbirth, when women report a broad spectrum of experiences. Thinking about other reproductive stages, such as adolescence or pregnancy, while these are defined primarily by the physical changes that are taking place, it is hard to separate out the other significant psycho-social changes that take place at the time. We would think about menopause in a similar way.

Women can often review their lives at this age and may have existential thoughts about the past and the future, which are of course quite normal. Whether these changes are experienced as a result of the menopause, or are linked to it, will vary between women and will in part be a function of what is happening in their lives, as well as the social and cultural meanings of ageing and menopause.

When does it happen and how long does it last?

Remember that the menopause can occur quite normally during a wide age range – at any time between 40 and 60 years, in fact. Studies have found that in some parts of the world, however, women experience the menopause slightly earlier. For example, in India and Pakistan, menopause age ranges from 44 to 48 years (average 47 years), compared with 50 to 51 in Europe and North America. Earlier menopause can be associated with poverty, poor nutrition and smoking (Freeman and Sherif 2007; Andrikoula and Prevelic 2009). Menopause is considered early, or premature, when it occurs in women aged 40 or younger, and this is estimated to affect approximately 1 per cent of women (Panay and Fenton 2008). The causes of early menopause are often unknown, but early menopause can be caused by certain genetic conditions, as well as some autoimmune disorders. Menopause also happens earlier due to surgery (surgical removal of the ovaries, or oophorectomy); medical treatments, such as chemotherapy and radiotherapy; or some hormone treatments, which interfere with natural hormone production. Medically induced menopause, if not caused by surgery, can be permanent or temporary. This can be the case for women who have had chemotherapy to treat breast cancer. So, if this has happened to you and you are uncertain about your menopausal status or fertility, do discuss this with your doctor.

If you have had a hysterectomy, you will not be having menstrual periods, and so it can be difficult to know when you have reached the menopause. If you still have ovaries, you will go through the menopause at roughly the same age as other women. However, you may have a slightly earlier menopause on average than those who have gone through this stage naturally. If you are having a hysterectomy, it is important to be clear about the difference between this operation (surgical removal of the womb) and surgical removal of the ovaries (oophorectomy) as the consequences are very different. Oophorectomy does cause menopause and rapid hormone changes, which can lead to more severe hot flushes if not treated. Women who have had surgical menopause and those who have early menopause are advised to use HRT until the natural age of menopause, i.e. 50 years, to maintain good health.

How long the menopause lasts is really very variable. Typically, it was thought to last between two and five years, but recent studies suggest that the duration of the menopause can be longer. In a 13-year Australian study (Col *et al.* 2009) following women through the menopause, the average duration (from the onset of menstrual changes to the stopping of hot flushes) was five to six years. But some women still have hot flushes and night sweats in their late 50s and early 60s (Hunter *et al.* 2012; Avis *et al.* 2015). This may be partly due to some women stopping HRT and having hot flushes later as their bodies adjust to the lowering of oestrogen levels.

Is there a male menopause?

The term 'male menopause' is often used in the media to explain a range of 'symptoms' experienced by middle-aged and older men, such as low libido, impotence, tiredness or depression. As for women, the term has negative connotations and is often used as a jokey insult. 'Male menopause' also suggests that the symptoms noted earlier occur as a result of a sudden drop in the hormone testosterone during middle age. This is not the case, however: testosterone levels reduce very gradually as men age, in fact, and the decline is steady at about 1 to 2 per cent each year from around the age of 40. Low levels of testosterone can sometimes be responsible for symptoms, but this is quite rare, affecting an estimated 2 per cent of men.

In most cases the symptoms are nothing to do with hormones, and, just as for women, lifestyle factors, age or stresses – such as work or relationship issues, divorce, money problems or ageing parents – are more likely causes (McKinlay *et al.* 2007). Similarly, midlife can be a time of anxiety about ageing and accomplishments. However, some men do have menopausal symptoms – hot flushes and night sweats, for example – if they have testosterone-reducing treatments for prostate cancer, and these symptoms can be embarrassing and uncomfortable (Eziefula *et al.* 2013; Hunter and Stefanopoulou 2016).

Why do we have menopause?

Human females are unusual in that their reproductive ageing happens on average well before other age-related physical changes. Most animals and birds continue to reproduce through-out life. Some animals, particularly non-human primates and animals such as elephants that have long lifespans (especially if living in captivity), have varying lengths of post-reproductive life. In general, however, amongst non-human primates, infer-tility is associated with advanced age. Even chimpanzees, our closest relative, reach this reproductive stage anytime between mid-age and death, depending on how long they live. So why are humans different in this respect? There are no definite answers, but two main theories have been proposed. These can be summarized as (i) non-adaptive theories (Finn 2002) and (ii) adaptive theories (Rashidi and Shanley 2009).

One theory suggests that the menopause happens because of two non-adaptive evolutionary developments. First, because we have a large but limited supply of eggs at birth, and sec-ond, because we have a considerably longer lifespan than other mammals of similar size. As a result, we run out of eggs by mid-age, at a time when other physical systems are ageing much more slowly.

In contrast 'adaptive' theories suggest that menopause offers benefits; for example, postmenopausal women avoid the dangers of childbirth, which are more common with increasing age. Other theories emphasize the role of the mother and the grandmother in supporting the next generations. The mother theory focuses on the unusually long duration of child devel-opment in humans – and therefore the time women need to raise children – which is much longer than for other animals. So women need an extra 15 years or so of life after their last child is born in order to nurture their offspring. The grand-mother theory emphasizes the evolutionary benefits of having a grandmother to assist mothers with childcare and the care of other children. It has even been suggested that the evolution of the menopause has been important in extending our lifespans due to increased support for younger generations and reduced reproductive costs: for example, those related to childcare. We still do not know for sure why we have menopause, but this latter theory in particular seems to suggest there are some benefits to it.

Biological changes

The menopause is triggered by hormone changes. However, hormone production is influenced by a complex system of interactions between the ovaries, our hormones and the brain

(Burger 2006), the hypothalamic-pituitary-ovarian axis. The main hormones produced by the ovary are oestrogen (oestradiol), progesterone and testosterone.

During the menstrual cycle, hormones are sent directly into the bloodstream from the ovaries, as well as from the adrenal glands (which are just above the kidneys). The pituitary gland at the base of the brain releases a follicle-stimulating hormone (FSH) and a luteinizing hormone (LH). FSH and LH cause the ovaries to release oestrogen and progesterone. In a feedback loop, the levels of oestrogen and progesterone in the bloodstream then regulate the amounts of FSH and LH that are produced. So during a regular menstrual cycle, this system adjusts and regulates the amounts of hormones in the body. During the first half of the menstrual cycle, FSH causes the egg (ovum) to develop and mature, and oestrogen levels rise. Ovulation (which occurs when the egg leaves the ovaries) is triggered when oestrogen reaches a certain level in the bloodstream, and this causes the pituitary to produce LH. If pregnancy does not occur, levels of oestrogen and progesterone fall, and the lining of the womb is shed. Menstruation occurs, and the whole cycle continues again.

Menopause occurs when the number of eggs (or follicles) within the ovaries falls below a certain level. While at birth there are approximately 700,000 follicles in a woman's ovaries, the numbers reduce markedly in the decade before the menopause, and at the time of the last menstrual period, few remain. As the menopause approaches, the feedback mechanism between the ovaries and the pituitary gland is upset. As a result, there is a gradual increase in circulating levels of FSH and (later) of LH; there is also a gradual decrease in levels of oestradiol (oestrogen) concentrations in the blood. It is as if these hormones are working overtime to try to trigger some activity from the ovaries. As the ovaries become less responsive, menstrual cycles become 'anovulatory' – in other words, do not contain any fertile eggs – and eventually menstrual periods stop. This happens in a range of different ways. Some women experience regular menstruation and then one final period before stopping altogether, but for most of us, periods will become irregular and unpredictable, gradually lessening in frequency over a period of time. They may also be heavier or lighter than normal as menopause approaches.

Do remember that sexually active women can still become pregnant for at least a year following their last menstrual period. Women are advised to use contraceptives for two years after the last menstrual period if under 50 years of age and one year if they are over 50.

During the reproductive years, oestradiol is the main type of oestrogen produced. After the menopause, oestrogen production does not stop completely because another oestrogen, oestrone, is produced from three main sources:

1 from the adrenal cortex in the adrenal gland;
2 indirectly from the body's fat cells, which convert another hormone (androstenedione) to oestrone; and
3 from the ovaries, which continue to produce small quantities of androgens, which are converted to oestrogens.

After the menopause, about 85 per cent of the oestrogens circulating in the bloodstream are produced by the adrenals and 15 per cent by the ovaries. Menopausal symptoms – hot flushes and night sweats – occur as a result of the lowering of oestrogen levels; when oestrogen levels stabilize at a lower level, then the symptoms also tend to stop.

Psycho-social and cultural factors

Having described the biological factors influencing menopause, we now move on to examine some of the historical and social factors that have given the menopause its social and cultural meanings. These meanings can influence how we view this key event in women's lives. In general, menopause has had bad press. There are several reasons for this, including a poor understanding of biological changes, negative attitudes to older women and medical approaches that treat menopause squarely as an 'illness' with a host of negative consequences.

Historical perspectives

Scientific and medical writings about menopause in the Western world have contributed to a stereotypically negative picture of the menopausal woman as irritable, depressed, asexual and besieged by hot flushes (Hunter and O'Dea 1997). Negative views of menopause date back at least as far as Roman times, when the menstrual cycle was not understood, and menstrual blood was seen as dangerous and poisonous (Wilbush 1979). Blood-letting, by cutting veins or applying leeches, was a common treatment used in an attempt to preserve well-being as well as physical and sexual attractiveness.

Menopausal complaints were first treated by doctors in 18th-century France (Wilbush 1979). During this time, economic conditions in Europe improved, and life expectancy rose. Psychiatric and gynaecological theories in the 19th century linked a woman's reproductive capacity with her emotional well-being and even her sanity. Expressions of distress or dissatisfaction could be seen as sexual or 'hysterical', in origin and gynaecological surgery, such as hysterectomy, was used as a treatment (Showalter 1987). Psychoanalytic theories promoted the menopause as a neurosis, in which women mourned their loss of femininity and sexuality (Deutsch 1945). Women's distress was, it seems, overly attributed to her reproductive cycle, and as a result any social and psychological causes may well have been ignored.

It was not until the 1920s that the main hormones produced by the ovaries were identified, and the biological aspects of the menopause transition became better understood. Oestrogen therapy was prescribed for menopausal symptoms during the 1940s and 50s in the United States, principally to tackle flushes and night sweats initially. At this time doctors tended to view the menopause as an 'oestrogen deficiency disease', rather than a normal phase of women's lives. For example, in his book *Feminine Forever* (1966), R. A. Wilson claimed that this 'youth pill' (oestrogen) could avert 26 psychological and physical complaints. The menopausal woman was viewed as 'an unstable, oestrogen-starved' woman who is responsible for 'untold misery of alcoholism, drug addiction, divorce and broken homes'. His book was a bestseller, and many women would have been exposed to descriptions such as, 'No woman can escape the horror of this living decay. . . . [E]ven the most valiant woman can no longer hide the fact that she is, in effect, no longer a woman' (Wilson 1966). This view is likely to have had a very negative impact on how mid-aged women were viewed. The promotion of HRT focused on a range of negative consequences of the menopause that the treatment would address, the message being that if you didn't use HRT, you would be unattractive, unhealthy and in a state of decline! Furthermore, it gave weight to the idea that declining levels of oestrogen were pathological (in other words, akin to an illness) rather than a normal part of life.

We would argue that an *overly* medical perspective is likely to reinforce negative views about menopause and ageing, which can in turn influence today's women in their beliefs and attitudes towards menopause. If a large section of the population is viewed as unstable or vulnerable, it can be dismissed as inferior and need not be taken seriously. Jokes and embarrassment can be a way of distancing ourselves from the discomfort of this image. Similarly, the focus on a 'sudden decline' and 'long-term' consequences for health is anxiety-provoking and might encourage women to find medical solutions to reduce this anxiety.

There have been – and still are – polarized and often extreme theories and approaches to menopause and mid-aged women, including gynaecological, psychiatric and feminist theories (Hunter and Rendall 2007). Each approach suggests different perspectives on menopause. So, while the biomedical perspective presents a negative view of menopausal women as in a state of decline, feminist perspectives focus on the menopause as a natural phase of life and emphasize the positive aspects of being an older woman, such as the freedom from traditional roles and wisdom. Similarly, there are contrasting beliefs about treatments for troublesome menopausal symptoms, such as HRT versus alternative approaches like herbal remedies. The woman herself is often left uncertain in the midst of conflicting information and advice.

On the positive side, there is now more of an acceptance of a bio-psycho-social perspective of the menopause, more women are talking about menopause and more research is being undertaken to develop new forms of HRT and safe non-hormonal treatments.

Cross-cultural perspectives

Many women in Western cultures report hot flushes, night sweats and tiredness during the menopause transition. But hot flushes and night sweats are not as widely reported in countries such as India, Japan and China (Freeman and Sherif 2007). Japanese women, for example, tend to report headaches, chilliness and shoulder stiffness as the most troublesome menopausal symptoms. Cross-cultural research is difficult to conduct, but there is increasing evidence that a range of factors, such as lifestyle (smoking, diet, exercise), reproductive history, social and economic factors, body mass index (BMI) and beliefs and attitudes towards menopause, might together explain cultural variations in experience of the menopause (Andrikoula and Prevelic 2009; Avis et al. 2001; Freeman and Sherif 2007; Melby et al. 2005). For example, Japanese women may report fewer hot flushes because they have a diet high in soy, which contains phytoestrogens (plant-derived oestrogens).

Anthropological studies of women living in different cultures have provided examples of how menopause can be a positive event for some women, particularly when it is associated with affirming changes in social roles and status (Flint 1975). Early studies suggest the benefits of menopause in some cultures include freedom from the social taboos and restrictions associated with menstruation, as well as a liberation from the burdens of repeated pregnancies. Pregnancy can be dangerous and stressful in some countries due to poor medical facilities (Beyene 1986). Furthermore, menopause in many developing countries tends not to be regarded as a medical problem and thus might be accepted more as a natural part of life, with less focus on 'symptoms'. In a more recent study comparing experiences of menopause amongst White Australian women and women in Laos, Australian women reported higher rates of depression, as well as fears of aging, weight gain and cancer – fears not reported by Laotian women, who positioned menopause as a positive event (Sayakhot et al. 2012).

There are cultural differences in the meanings of the menopause, as well as the attributions of different types of symptoms to the menopause. For example, in a study of Asian women and White British women living in the UK and Asian women living in Delhi, a range of different consequences of the menopause were mentioned. For example:

> Relief from dirt, mess, embarrassment, need for sanitary protection, heavy periods. Can go to the temple, do prayers, not interrupt religious activities.

> You can't have children, not a problem; I already have children; it [is] a good thing–I have so many.

> When periods stop, health becomes bad; affects eyes and whole body; causes illness.

However, in general the menopause was viewed as a normal part of life despite its differing consequences.

> No difference; a natural thing; it is the cycle of life; accept it; it has to happen.

> I don't mind; it doesn't bother me. . . . [P]art of life; life just goes on.

All three groups of women shared the view that the menopause does not necessarily cause major changes, that it is a relief to stop having menstrual periods and that the menopause is a marker of ageing. However, while the Asian women also welcomed the benefits of having no periods (relief of embarrassment and greater religious freedoms), they also associated the cessation of periods with poor health and illness. Both groups of Asian women commonly attributed ocular changes (becoming short-sighted in middle age) to the menopause, as well as weight gain and high blood pressure; the white British women reported tiredness and mood changes as a result of the menopause, in addition to hot flushes (Gupta *et al*. 2006a; Hunter *et al*. 2009c).

In most cultures, and particularly in Western societies, women tend to be valued for their physical and sexual attractiveness, reproductive capacity and youthfulness. Negative attitudes to ageing are common. In addition, there is a general belief, probably influenced by historical meanings, that women going through menopause inevitably become depressed and age more rapidly, yet there is no conclusive evidence to support this (Dennerstein *et al*. 2004; Mishra and Kuh 2012). It is interesting to note that younger women tend to have more negative attitudes to the menopause than older women who have actually experienced it (Smith *et al*. 2011; Brown *et al*. 2017). For women who have been through this transition, the menopause can seem less important than it did when they were younger, especially now that women today are likely to live for several decades after this (typically) midlife event:

> Well, I have to say that now I am in my 60s and look back, the menopause is not a big deal. . . . [I]n fact my younger friends are now going through it and these days for me 50 is really not old.

There is some evidence that very negative attitudes and expectations before the menopause are associated with a more difficult experience of menopause (Ayers *et al*. 2010). For example, in two studies, women were followed through the menopause transition; those who had more negative attitudes about menopause beforehand were more likely to report depressed mood and other symptoms during the menopause, suggesting that negative attitudes towards menopause can affect symptom experience – in effect, a self-fulfilling prophecy (Avis and McKinlay 1991; Avis *et al*. 1997). This is perhaps not too surprising, however, since if we think that we are going to become 'unattractive, over-emotional and prone to long-term illness' this might well affect how we feel. Therefore, menopause (cessation of menstruation) is a fairly universal event, but the meaning of the menopause and how it is experienced varies considerably within and across cultures. For many women, menopause is a time for reflection.

A time of decline or a positive life stage?

In the past 20 years, several studies have been published that help to clarify what women really do experience during the menopause. Does it represent a time of decline, or could it be a positive life stage? We will describe these studies, each of which ask women about their own personal experience of menopause. We also include brief summaries of research findings on mood and quality of life, sexual functioning, weight, memory and osteoporosis and where relevant 'menopause myths' are challenged.

Mood and quality of life during the menopause

Investigating relationships between menopause and mood or quality of life has been a difficult area to research, and longitudinal studies that follow women through the menopause transition have been designed to specifically address this issue (Avis *et al.* 2003; Dennerstein *et al.* 2004; Kuh *et al.* 1997; Woods *et al.* 2005, 2006). The main findings from these studies suggest that the menopause transition is not directly associated with depression or reduced quality of life for most women.

Two studies provide important results: the first (Lang *et al.* 2011) used data from the Household Survey for England study of 94,879 men and women and investigated psychological distress across age bands in both genders. The authors found an increase in distress in the age bands 35 to 54 for men and women and an improvement in mood after the age of 55. This increase in depressed mood during the 'midlife' or the 'reproductive years' has been found in previous studies and has been ascribed to women's hormones – and also to the 'male menopause'. However, when the researchers divided the men and women into different levels of socioeconomic status (based on income), they found that the increase in distress during midlife occurred only for those women and men who were in the lowest 20 per cent of the income bands. These results certainly show the impact of social and economic factors upon well-being. The reproductive years tend to be the years during which both men and women may be engaged with work, child-rearing and other responsibilities. When asked about life pressures that impact on quality of life, men and women in their 40s and early 50s tend to cite work, health, financial and family problems as the main stresses (O'Dea *et al.* 1999).

Another take-home message from the study by Lang *et al.* is that mood tends to improve for women after the menopause – there may be some truth, therefore, in the idea of 'postmenopause zest'! Some women do have more time for themselves after the menopause and are able to pursue new interests. In another study, interviews with women over a five-year period throughout the menopause transition revealed that as menopause progressed, the majority of women tended to develop more positive views of menopause, and these changes were associated with reports of newfound freedom and personal growth (Busch *et al.* 2003). Campbell *et al.* (2017) interviewed women over a 20-year period and found an improvement in mood postmenopause, and in general it is recognised that emotional well-being improves with age as people tend to become more equable and self-assured (Parry 2017).

There are however considerable differences between people in terms of life circumstances. Each generation of women may differ in their experience of menopause and midlife because of environmental and social factors that have influenced them throughout their lives. These days, women in their 50s are likely to have very different lifestyles in comparison with their mothers at the same age. They have social media and the internet; they are more likely to be working outside the home; some might be starting new jobs, interests or relationships, for example, while others might have grandchildren or might be in the throes of bringing up adolescent children. The 'empty nest syndrome' that might have occurred for women in their early 50s in the past, now does not necessarily happen at, or coincide with, menopause. Research conducted on the effects of children leaving home suggests that this is not usually a traumatic event although it can, like most life transitions, bring both positive and negative impacts, such as a spare room and/or missing the company of a son or daughter. However, the fact that today many 'children' are still living at home well into their 20s because of financial pressures means that midlife can be a period during which children remain financially dependent, while parents, now often living until their 80s or even 90s, need to be cared for longer.

The second study is the Medical Research Council National Survey of Health and Development. The authors, Mishra and Kuh (2012), investigated 695 women followed up regularly since birth in 1946 and every year between the ages of 47 and 54. The women in the study all experienced natural menopause (i.e. did not have a medically or surgically induced menopause) and reported on their health and well-being. In this well-conducted study, four groups of symptoms reported by the women were examined over time: psychological, physical and vasomotor (hot flushes and night sweats) and sexual functioning.

The results were as follows:

- **Psychological symptoms.** 77 per cent of the women experienced no change across the menopause transition; 10 per cent had an increase in psychological symptoms which coincided with the menopause and reduced two to three years afterwards; 13 per cent had symptoms which improved across the menopause transition.
- **Physical symptoms.** Overall, these showed no relationship with the menopause transition.
- **Vasomotor symptoms (hot flushes and night sweats).** 49 per cent experienced very mild symptoms which showed a small increase during the menopause transition; 26 per cent experienced moderate symptoms, mainly in the postmenopause period; 14 per cent had moderate to severe symptoms, mainly in the early transition; 11 per cent had more severe symptoms that continued for up to four years after the menopause (the study did not have information after the age of 54 years).
- **Sexual functioning.** 70 per cent of the women reported no or very mild discomfort; 7 per cent reported more severe discomfort, but this was not specifically associated with menopause stages; 12 per cent reported improvements and 10 per cent had more sexual discomfort after the menopause.

Taken together these results show that, overall, general physical symptoms are not particularly linked to the menopause transition and that about 10 per cent have significant psychological symptoms (such as depressed mood and anxiety) that are associated with the timing of the menopause. For these women, psychological symptoms tend to occur during the perimenopause, when hormone levels are changing, and hot flushes are common.

Depressed mood and anxiety can certainly occur during the menopause transition as during other life stages, and it can be difficult to pinpoint the causes when there is so much going on. It is easy to attribute low moods and anxieties to the hormones and the menopause, but there are often other causes.

There are complex and bidirectional relationships between hot flushes and low mood (Maki *et al.* 2019). Depression is common, with about 20 per cent of the population likely to experience significant depression at some stage of their lives. It is also a normal reaction to loss and happens when we adjust to life changes. There is a difference between depressed mood, which is even more common and quite normal, and severe or clinical depression, which typically requires some professional help (see Chapter 3). However, moderate to severe depression is usually more likely to be associated with life difficulties – such as ill health, chronic social problems and losses and a past history of depression – than with specific hormonal changes.

The main factors influencing depressed mood during the menopause include:

- problematic hot flushes and night sweats that affect daily activity and sleep;
- your general self-esteem – self-esteem can develop across the course of our lives but is often more closely linked to what we think about ourselves than external factors (see Fennell 2016);
- life stresses, such as problems at work, financial problems, worries regarding children or caring for parents and relationship problems; and
- social support, such as having friends, family or a confidant, which acts like a buffer against stress.

Studies pulling together the research to try and tease out the links between menopause and mood have identified that while most women are OK, there are risk factors that make mood issues more likely, and these are not necessarily related to the hormonal changes of menopause. Overall, women are more likely to experience mood issues during menopause if they have a history of depression, post-natal depression or premenstrual mood issues; are experiencing significant stresses or life events as stated earlier; have negative beliefs about menopause and aging; or have had a surgical menopause (Vivian-Taylor and Hickey 2014). Having persistent and/or troublesome hot flushes and sleep problems can also make women feel depressed and irritable. Hot flushes and night sweats can also lead to considerable anxiety as they make our bodies feel out of control, and they can cause rapid heartbeats, or palpitations, which are similar to anxiety reactions. Unexpected flushes can also cause anxiety. In turn, stress can influence hormone levels as well, meaning that there can be interactions between stress, hormone levels and hot flushes. The combination of life stress, low mood and anxiety can make menopausal symptoms worse, and intrusive menopausal symptoms exacerbate mood issues and general stress, setting up a vicious cycle.

For some women tension or low mood during the perimenopause is often described in ways that are similar to premenstrual mood changes, such as extra sensitivity, having 'mood swings' or feeling rather vulnerable or 'flat'.

My face changes and I have less energy, I feel easily overwhelmed and over-reactive to situations that normally I can deal with. It seems to come on around my periods but it is unpredictable and that's half the problem.

For the women who have this pattern, these symptoms are likely to stop when hormone changes settle down towards the end of the menopause transition (Vivian-Taylor and Hickey 2014)

The menopause is often associated with uncertainty – partly because what women experience varies considerably, from when it occurs to how long it lasts and whether there are troublesome symptoms or not. An early menopause can be distressing due to its impact on fertility and concerns about health and fears of rapid ageing following early menopause, drawing upon the negative stereotypes described earlier (Singer et al. 2011). Early menopause that is induced by breast cancer treatments can feel like the last straw when menopausal symptoms are felt at a time when women are trying to get their lives back to normal (Parton et al. 2017).

Uncertainty can be anxiety provoking especially if we fear the worst – for example, if we think we will age dramatically or virtually overnight, we are likely to find the transition a particularly daunting prospect. It helps to have a balanced view, and one of our aims with this book is to help you to develop this through information and cognitive behavioural strategies. Encouragingly, it has been shown that emotional happiness and life satisfaction with factors such as work, family and health can be protective factors that enable women to weather the storms that the menopause can present (Brown et al. 2015). The self-help guide will help you to think about how to prioritise enjoyable and meaningful activities within your current situation alongside the other CBT strategies aimed at reducing distress.

Sexual health and menopause

The results for sexual discomfort identify a link with the timing of menopause. The likelihood of vaginal dryness (less lubrication; dryness; and, for some, painful intercourse) increases across the menopausal transition. Vaginal dryness and discomfort are associated with the lower oestrogen levels and occur more frequently in the postmenopause phase. For more information see: www.womens-health-concern.org/wp-content/uploads/2018/03/WHC-FACTSHEET-VaginalDryness-MAR2018.pdf.

Lubricants, moisturisers and local vaginal oestrogen can be helpful; moisturisers and lubricants that have ingredients that match women's natural secretions are more comfortable and are now recommended (Edwards and Panay 2016). Some examples are included in Box 1.2.

Box 1.2 There are specific medical options for vaginal dryness and painful sex, if this is a problem.

- Vaginal lubricants can reduce discomfort with sexual activity and are available without a prescription. They are designed to have short-term effects and to be used to make sexual activity more comfortable, e.g. Sylk, Yes, Pjurmed.
- Vaginal moisturisers line the wall of the vagina and maintain vaginal moisture. These are used two to three times a week, are designed to have positive and longer-lasting general effects on vaginal tissue and are available at pharmacists and on prescription, e.g. Replens, YesVM, Regelle.
- Regular sexual stimulation promotes blood flow and secretions to the vagina.
- Pelvic floor exercises can tone pelvic floor muscles.
- Vaginal oestrogen therapy in the form of low-dose local oestrogen, applied directly to the vagina, can be an effective treatment for vaginal dryness and discomfort during sexual activity. It is available on prescription, so do discuss it with your doctor although is generally not recommended for women who have a history of breast cancer.

For women with a history of breast cancer, non-hormonal moisturisers are recommended as the first line of choice and for intercourse specifically, paraben-free vaginal moisturisers with acidic PH, in line with WHO recommendations (Sassarini *et al.* 2018).

Sexual interest in general tends to reduce with age and across the menopause transition, but this has been found to be associated with a range of factors. These include sexual functioning before the menopause, stress, ill health, problematic hot flushes and night sweats, low mood, relationship status (being in a relationship or having a new partner), a partner's sexual functioning, attitudes towards sex and ageing and cultural background (including beliefs about the importance of sex) (Avis *et al.* 2000, 2005). Overall, previous sexual functioning and relationship factors seem to be more important influences on women's sexual lives during the menopause than hormonal factors (Dennerstein *et al.* 2005).

It is also important to remember that not all women or men are sexually active. Despite changes in some aspects of sexual functioning with age and menopause, many women who are in relationships report being satisfied with their sexual relationships. For example, people often make adjustments in response to their circumstances, such as ill health, and maintain intimacy in their relationships (Ussher *et al.* 2013).

> Starting a new relationship at this age, in my 50s, made me a bit worried – I hadn't had a relationship since my divorce eight years ago and didn't know how I would respond. It was a bit tricky at first but he was so relaxed. . . . [N]ow we are fine. My friend recommended lubricants that helped too.

> Having breast cancer made me think [that] sex isn't the most important thing at this stage. . . . [M]y health is the main thing. I'm just going to wait and see how I feel. . . . [T]here's no pressure.

Therefore, as well as the medical approaches described in Box 1.2, there are things to consider if this is a concern for you based on recent research. For example, using the self-help book to consider ways to manage and reduce stress such as relaxation, communicating with your partner and thinking together about what changes may be needed to adapt to your current situation can also be helpful. Winterich (2003) found that the women with active and fulfilling sex lives tended to communicate openly and were willing to change their sexual repertoire if needed to adapt to menopausal changes. Given the influence of negative attitudes to sex and aging, use the cognitive work in the stress section of the self-help guide to identify and address any negative assumptions about sex or any tendency to be self-critical within a sexual context. Together with the biomedical approaches, these strategies can help work towards a more fulfilling sex life.

Weight gain?

Weight gain is often a concern for women during and after the menopause.

Will I put on weight and develop 'middle-age spread'?

The steady weight gain of about 0.5 kg annually amongst women is largely due to age and associated lifestyle factors such as diet and lack of exercise (Davis *et al*. 2012). However, reduced oestrogen levels during menopause can lead to the redistribution of body fat. Women tend to find that their body shape may change as 'childbearing' fat moves from their hips and thighs, where it is no longer needed, to their stomach and middle. Abdominal fat is less healthy than fat on the hips, though, another reason for adopting a healthy diet and regular exercise. This does not seem to happen to everyone, and while some women do not like this change, others welcome it.

> I was always a typical pear shape and couldn't get jeans to look good on me. But now I can so this has been a bonus for me but some of my friends complain about having more fat around the waist.

For breast cancer patients, there are additional challenges as chemotherapy can lead to weight gain due to reduced activity levels and fatigue; medications such as steroids can lead to metabolic and appetite changes, cravings and comfort eating (American Society of Clinical Oncology 2019).

There are, however, steps to take to manage this change:

- Manage what you eat and how much you eat – in other words, eat well. Some foods and eating patterns increase weight gain, such as irregular eating habits and eating processed foods, desserts, sugary drinks and fried foods.
- Take regular exercise and keep active: for example, taking brisk walks, taking the stairs instead of the lift or walking to the shops instead of driving. The main thing is to find an exercise or activity that you enjoy. Going along to a class or activity with a friend can help make exercise more enjoyable and may increase the likelihood of attending even when you don't feel like it!

There is evidence to suggest that a weight-loss strategy that combines a healthy diet and exercise can lead to improvements in quality of life and also to improvements in hot flushes (Davis *et al.* 2012). A recent randomised controlled trial found that resistance training three times a week reduced the frequency of hot flushes by 50 per cent in (postmenopausal) women who previously had a sedentary lifestyle compared to a control group who did not change their activity level (Berin *et al.* 2019).

Exercise can also help improve sleep quality and reduce the time taken to fall asleep, particularly if done in the morning. Tworoger *et al.* (2004) divided sedentary postmenopausal women not taking HRT into four groups: two groups did moderate-intensity aerobic exercise for at least 45 minutes per day, and two other groups did a low-intensity stretching and relaxation exercise class for a similar duration. The groups were further divided into morning and evening exercisers. They found that women who exercised in the morning reported less trouble falling asleep, regardless of which exercise they did. Importantly, only those who did at least three hours a week reported this improvement.

Memory and menopause

Complaints about forgetfulness and poor memory are very common during midlife, and there is also concern about dementia, given its prevalence now that people are living longer.

> My mother has dementia and it does worry me – I am much more aware if I can't remember names of films or acquaintances.

> All my friends at work are about my age and we just laugh about it – I remember the important things. I think that there is just too much information and it is easy to expect ourselves to remember everything.

Despite many women reporting difficulties with memory during menopause, there is very little evidence that any decline in memory is solely due to it. Studies have concluded that both men and women show some age-related memory changes (Singh-Manoux *et al.* 2012). In fact, there is research evidence showing that reports of memory problems are more strongly associated with stress and mood than with hormone levels or stage of menopause (Mitchell and Woods 2011). In addition, subjective reports of memory problems during midlife are not necessarily associated with objective memory performance measured by tests of memory (Henderson 2009). This is reassuring because if people worry about not being able to remember, it can make the situation worse. Nevertheless, women often say that they have 'brain fog', which could be caused by multiple factors – including sleep disruption, stress and hormone fluctuations. Breast cancer patients tend to report memory problems with low to moderate doses of chemotherapy, which tend to improve over time once chemotherapy is completed (Falleti *et al.* 2005).

Studies of HRT have not proved that HRT helps memory or prevents dementia. It is possible that there is a 'window of opportunity' for HRT to have beneficial results and few side effects if used only for younger women for a short time, but more research is needed (NICE 2015b). Advice from the North American Menopause Society states that on the basis of the evidence, they do not recommend HRT for the sole prevention of cognitive ageing or dementia (Utian 2008).

There are steps you can take if you find yourself having too much to remember. It can help to be aware of situations in which you are prone to forgetting or being distracted – for example, when you are tired, stressed at work or at the end of the day – and preparing for these in advance: for example, with a 'schedule' or rehearsal. Stress can have an impact on memory, so anything that reduces it, such as doing one thing at a time, should help to improve attention and memory. And don't worry too much or try too hard if you can't remember something!

Ferguson *et al.* (2007) developed a CBT-orientated self-help intervention for breast cancer patients experiencing memory problems following chemotherapy that contains helpful ideas that you can practise yourself. They found that relaxation training, pleasant activity scheduling and specific memory strategies such as verbal rehearsal (repeating something silently to yourself such as a phone number or an everyday task), linking an image to something you needed to remember and making a schedule for regular tasks all led to significant improvements in memory two months later, and the improvements were maintained after six months. Furthermore, the women involved in the study reported an improvement in quality of life.

Osteoporosis

The menopause is often associated in people's minds with osteoporosis to the extent that you might think that you will develop osteoporosis just because you have entered menopause. This is not the case. Osteoporosis is an age-related condition characterized by decreased bone mass and increased susceptibility to bone fractures. It affects men, too, but it is more common among older women. Bone is built up during childhood, adolescence and young adult life, usually reaching maximum thickness in our early thirties. Oestrogen levels do have an impact on bone mass, because oestrogen slows down bone re-absorption, so after the menopause, there is a slight decrease in bone mass. However, osteoporosis is an acceleration of bone loss that typically leads to fractures in our 70s and 80s. It also tends to run in families. There are a number of factors that are linked to its development, and osteoporosis is increasing due to longer life expectancy but also as a result of lifestyle factors such as exercise and diet.

There are a number of ways to prevent osteoporosis. Having a good calcium intake is important, as is taking regular weight-bearing exercise and cutting back on smoking, alcohol and caffeine. These measures are helpful at any age but are particularly crucial for children and young women, as they will help maximize peak bone mass. Early menopause is a risk factor, so if you have a menopause before the age of 45, it is advisable to discuss HRT to protect the bones with your doctor. In order to minimize bone loss during and after the menopause, a good calcium intake is again recommended, as is exercise such as dancing, brisk walking or jogging (North American Menopause Society 2010). There is also evidence that increasing exercise levels significantly improves bone density in older people (Marques *et al*. 2012).

Bone mineral density testing (most often with a DEXA scan) measures the thickness of the bone, usually in the hip and spine. This test can help to diagnose bone loss and predict a person's risk of future bone fractures. Bisphosphonates are the main drugs used to prevent and treat osteoporosis in postmenopausal women, and they help reduce loss and further thinning of the bone. Hormone replacement therapy (HRT) can prevent bone loss in younger postmenopausal women, and the benefits continue while taking HRT but decrease once treatment is stopped (NICE 2015b). Other new therapies for osteoporosis are currently being developed. For further information, contact the National Osteoporosis Society and British Menopause Society (in Resources).

Women's accounts of menopause

Let's look now at what women themselves say about menopause – is it a time of crisis, loss or decline? A medical problem? Or a new phase offering liberation and new life choices? Studies based on in-depth interviews with women tend to show that, overall, menopause is not viewed as negatively as you might expect.

Women's accounts typically include both positive and negative aspects at the same time, such as relief from cessation of menstrual periods and the risk of pregnancy, but also concerns about ageing and negative images of the menopause (Hunter and O'Dea 1997; Hvas 2006; Perz and Ussher 2008). For example, in a recent UK study, three interrelated narratives of menopause emerged from the accounts of 48 midlife women: (i) menopause as a normal, biological process distinct from self, identity and social transitions; (ii) menopause as a struggle provoking distress and a time of identity loss and social upheaval; and (iii) menopause as a time of liberation and transformation (de Salis *et al.* 2018). Related themes (e.g., dealing with negative stereotypes of women's aging, expectations and uncertainties about future physical and emotional problems, taboos and silence, relief, reflection and growth) have been previously reported (Hunter and O'Dea 1997; Hvas 2006; Rubinstein and Foster 2013; Sergeant and Rizq 2017).

We interviewed 50 British women and asked about their experiences and beliefs about menopause (Hunter and O'Dea 1997; Hunter *et al.* 1997). Overall, the women tended to view it as a natural process that generally did not require medical intervention; however, in certain circumstances – for example, if women had problematic hot flushes or night sweats – it might then be viewed as a medical problem. So, this view of the menopause was flexible and a reasonable reaction to the experience of the menopause that, as we have shown, differs considerably between women. The interviewees also reported a range of positive, neutral and negative experiences and reactions. For example, there was an expectation and awareness of change.

I didn't like my periods being irregular or my body feeling different but in myself, well, I still felt that inside I hadn't changed.

Women reported that they were pleased that they no longer had to deal with periods, premenstrual problems or fear of pregnancy, suggesting menopause was in part a relief rather than a sense of loss.

> It's nice to get it over with and not have periods any more.

> I was a person who suffered an awful lot with my periods and it stopped me doing a lot of things when I was younger. . . . [B]ut now I've lost all that, which is beautiful!

Most women were fairly neutral about the ending of reproductive capacity (fertility), feeling that this had been dealt with in the previous 10 or 15 years – this was, however, likely to be more of an issue for women who experienced early menopause or who have had fertility problems.

> I never really wanted to have children so it never worried me in that regard. I'll be quite pleased in some ways.

> It gives you the feeling [that] it's the end of something, your reproductive time. But I mean, I think that ended a little time ago. I wouldn't have dreamed of having a baby after 45, so I'm not looking for that.

They also spoke about dealing with hot flushes and night sweats, which affected their lives to differing degrees.

> I get hot at times but it doesn't bother me. If it's hot, I just open the window but otherwise I don't have any ill effects at all.

> You can actually feel the sweat trickling down your head when you wake up during the night and then you're tired the next day, desperately [so] because you can't sleep. . . . I don't think people realise what an awful nuisance it is, because they think it's just an inconvenience.

And, perhaps not surprisingly, becoming older and passing their landmark 50th birthday were not generally welcomed; neither were the anticipated consequences of ageing. But some of these perceptions are likely to be overly negative: healthy women in their 50s and 60s are able to participate in full lives and do not age overnight on becoming menopausal!

> It brings home to you that perhaps you're in the last half of life. It's a time for a bit of reflection about where you're going over the next few years.

Finally, a common theme was a concern about the unknown and a fear of 'falling apart' and 'letting yourself go' during the menopause, which appeared to draw on negative social and historical beliefs of 'decline and decay'.

> You have to put yourself in order as well because when you go through something like that you become [sic] as though you are not interested in yourself – like you want to let yourself go.

One woman, recently married with a young daughter, described how her image of a menopausal woman did not fit within the context of her current life. Taking HRT was seen to be a way of resolving this conflict.

> I don't know because I'm staving it off. Well, I feel OK about myself, it's what other people need from me that's the difficulty. It's how I have to be as a wife and a mother to a young child. I've got to be there and . . . in action . . . so I've staved off the menopause for a while so that I can hold it all together.

This study shows how historical and cultural beliefs might subtly impact on personal concerns and reactions during the menopause: for example, the idea of falling apart, rapidly ageing or letting yourself go. Similarly, we have seen from cross-cultural studies that the ways in which older women are viewed and treated in different societies are likely to have an impact on attitudes to ageing. So women not only have to cope with a raft of physical changes, but they must face these negative stereotypes and media images too. Our study and that of Perz and Ussher (2008) found that, on the whole, women do find ways to negotiate and resist overly negative discourses of the menopause and are able to reach more balanced perspectives, particularly if they can share their views with others.

As we have learned, a range of positive, neutral and negative images of menopause was described by most women. What do you think about the menopause and your own experience?

What do you think about your menopause?

Positive consequences: --

Neutral consequences: --

Negative consequences: ---

In summary, the menopause is a bio-psycho-social life transition. Individual experiences vary greatly, so it is quite likely that when talking to others you will find that your own personal experience may not be the same as that of the next person. And there are many influences upon how we go through menopause, most of which we have little control over. So if you are having a challenging time, do not blame yourself. Instead, check that you are doing everything you can to help yourself through this stage of life. In the next chapter, the focus is specifically on the most common menopausal symptoms – hot flushes and night sweats.

2

Menopausal symptoms
Hot flushes and night sweats

What are hot flushes?

Hot flushes and night sweats are typically described as sensations of intense heat, accompanied by sweating and sometimes shivering and palpitations (rapid heartbeats). They are also called 'vasomotor' symptoms because they are associated with changes in the vascular system that affect blood flow in the body; for example, when hot flushes occur, there is an initial (vaso) dilation and subsequent (vaso)constriction of blood vessels. The sensations of heat and flushing of the skin typically occur in the face, neck and chest and can spread through the body. Women's experience of hot flushes and night sweats varies considerably, but these symptoms can disrupt daily life and sleep and consequently can affect quality of life (Ayers and Hunter 2012).

I can be at work or at home and then it happens – a sudden flash of heat across my back, neck and face and then I'm dripping with sweat. My face goes red and I just want to disappear.

Mine are worse at night. I just settle to try to go to sleep and then it comes over me. I feel hot and start to sweat. I have to get up and cool down in the bathroom, drinking cool water, and sometimes if it's really bad I'll change my nightclothes. I have to have the window open and no heating in the winter. It can take me a while to get back to sleep especially if I have woken up properly and start thinking.

The worst part of it for me is having flushes at work; if I'm in a meeting or in a rush I'm more likely to have one. I dread to think what my colleagues are thinking. I feel horrible sweating in the office and they must think I'm really embarrassed or anxious about something.

Although they can be similar in appearance to blushing, hot flushes have different physiological causes. Blushing is an emotional reaction associated with the release of adrenaline, which causes vasodilation of the blood vessels in the face (Hanisch *et al.* 2008).

What causes hot flushes?

It is generally understood that the rate of change of oestrogen (i.e. oestrogen withdrawal), rather than lower circulating oestrogen levels, leads to hot flushes and night sweats. For example, these symptoms are more severe amongst women who undergo surgical menopause (removal of the ovaries, or oophorectomy), resulting in rapid oestrogen withdrawal, and also following some medical treatments which reduce oestrogen levels, such as chemotherapy or hormone treatment for breast cancer. Although the exact causes of hot flushes and night sweats are not fully understood, the way that oestrogen withdrawal triggers them appears to occur centrally in a region of the brain that regulates temperature, the hypothalamus.

Oestrogen withdrawal is thought to reset the central temperature control system – a bit like changing the thermostat on the central heating (Archer *et al.* 2011). Normally, body temperature is maintained within a 'thermoneutral zone' (TNZ), which is a range of temperatures within which core body temperature varies without having to actively regulate itself. If core body temperature rises too much, for example, we self-regulate by sweating, which reduces our temperature to within the TNZ (Freedman and Krell 1999).

Based on laboratory studies of women experiencing hot flushes, Freedman (2005) found that women with hot flushes have a narrowed TNZ compared with women who do not (see Figure 2.1). Because of this, hot flushes can be triggered by small increases in core body temperature, which can be caused by changes in ambient temperature or triggers such as rushing or even caffeine. We then sweat or try to cool down when faced with small temperature changes in the environment. The hot flushes and night sweats are actually self-cooling mechanisms employed by our bodies to maintain body temperature within the normal range or TNZ (Figure 2.1). Consequently, while most women have hot flushes, others can also experience shivers or 'cold flushes'.

Noradrenaline and serotonin are substances known as neurotransmitters, and they are also involved in the physiology of

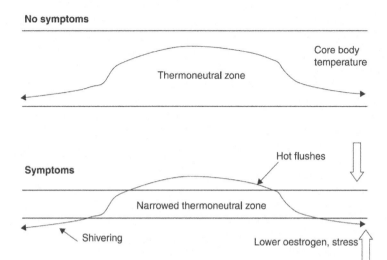

Figure 2.1 The thermoneutral zone (TNZ) and hot flushes: showing core
body temperature fluctuations within the TNZ for women
without hot flushes (no symptoms) and the narrowed TNZ for
women with hot flush symptoms

Source: Adapted and reproduced with kind permission from Archer *et al.*
(2011)

hot flushes and night sweats. There is some evidence that the
TNZ is narrowed by elevated brain noradrenaline. The roles
of oestrogen, noradrenaline and serotonin in hot flushes and
night sweats, although not fully understood, provide a ration-
ale for the use of oestrogen or HRT as well as selective serotonin reuptake inhibitors (SSRIs – antidepressants that are
prescribed for depression but also for hot flushes) in the management of these symptoms (see page 65).

Hot flushes are also associated with general stress and
anxiety (Slade and Amaee 1995; Woods *et al.* 2005; Freeman
et al. 2005) and can themselves result in social embarrassment and discomfort, whereas night sweats tend to be associated with sleep problems and tiredness. We also know that
stress produces changes in noradrenaline and serotonin, which
may affect the temperature control system in women with
hot flushes and night sweats. In one study of women experiencing hot flushes (Swartzman *et al.* 1990), more hot flushes
were reported when women were doing stressful tasks, such

as mental arithmetic, than when they were involved in calm or non-stressful tasks such as reading. The authors concluded that stress appears to narrow the TNZ, making the symptoms more likely to occur.

Specific triggers of hot flushes and night sweats can also be identified, but not all flushes have a specific trigger, and many simply come on without any warning. Certain situations – such as hot, crowded places; work meetings; enclosed spaces; and activities such as rushing, physical exertion or eating and drinking – have been reported to precipitate or exacerbate hot flushes, however (Gannon *et al.* 1987; Hunter and Liao 1995).

While night sweats are generally less frequent than hot flushes, they can be harder to tolerate because of their impact on sleep quality and daytime tiredness (Sievert *et al.* 2006). Sleep disruption is reported by approximately a quarter of menopausal women. A recent study of sleep across stages of the menopause found that sleep problems were associated with a range of factors including stress, night sweats, alcohol use, mood, age and health (Woods and Mitchell 2010). So sleep problems have other causes but are more common in women who experience frequent night sweats (Eichling *et al.* 2005).

How common are they?

Menopausal hot flushes and/or night sweats are reported by approximately 60 to 70 per cent of menopausal women in Western cultures (Freeman and Sherif 2007). In general, reporting of hot flushes and night sweats increases as women transition between early and late menopause. The frequency of bothersome hot flushes generally begins to rise two years before the last menstrual period and reaches its peak up to two years after the final menstrual period. There then tends to be a gradual decrease in subsequent postmenopausal years. However, there are considerable variations and different patterns between women; recent research suggests that some women tend to have flushes earlier in the menopause transition, while others have them later (Freeman, Sammel *et al.* 2011). Although it makes sense to view these symptoms as part of normal development during the menopause, given how often they occur, they are problematic for some women: approximately 25 per cent of menopausal women seek help for troublesome hot flushes and/ or night sweats.

Can we predict who will have troublesome hot flushes?

It is important to remember that there is marked variation between women in the duration, severity and frequency of hot flushes and night sweats experienced during menopause. It is also very difficult to predict who will have hot flushes and for most women, it is just bad luck – so it is important not to blame yourself if you do experience these symptoms. However, we hope to be able to provide some strategies for you to use to manage them, whatever their cause.

There is evidence that women who have had a surgical menopause (removal of ovaries) and/or a hysterectomy and women who have had breast cancer treatments are more likely to have troublesome hot flushes and night sweats. In addition, women who smoke cigarettes and who have low general levels of physical activity may be more likely to have problematic hot flushes (Ford et al. 2005; Hunter et al. 2012; Ziv-Gal and Flaws 2010). In general, research following large numbers of women both before and during the menopause transition suggest that those with higher levels of anxiety prior to the menopause (Freeman et al. 2005) and those under higher levels of stress during the menopause tend to report more troublesome hot flushes and night sweats (Hunter et al. 2009c, 2012). While they are still difficult to predict in individual cases – and of course it is impossible to change past events – there may be some practical things that you can change to reduce the impact of hot flushes. Giving up smoking, reducing stress and taking increased moderate physical activity would all be helpful, and all would be recommended for general health and well-being too.

The association between body weight or body mass index (BMI) and hot flushes remains unclear, but there are two conflicting theories on this subject. One suggests that women with more body fat, and therefore higher levels of circulating oestrogen, will have fewer hot flushes. The other suggests that women with higher BMIs would have more hot flushes because body fat tends to reduce heat loss. Heavier women might have more 'insulation', making it difficult for them to lose heat, which could lead to more hot flushes as the body tries to cool itself down.

Overall, there is more evidence to support the second theory associating heavier weight, and also weight gains during midlife, with more hot flushes (Gold et al. 2006; Thurston et al.

2008). For example, the prevalence and severity of hot flushes have been found to be associated specifically with weight increases, particularly around the waist (which can be estimated by increased waist circumference) during midlife (Li *et al*. 2003; Thurston *et al*. 2009). In a study of women across the UK, we found a small association between increases in waist size during adulthood and troublesome hot flushes (Hunter *et al*. 2012). On a practical level, hot flushes and night sweats might well be more uncomfortable and socially embarrassing for women who are heavier (Hunter and Haqqani 2011).

> After going through breast cancer treatment, I know I have put weight on. It's difficult because I still feel quite tired in the day so it's hard to exercise like I used to. Also I feel more embarrassed when I have the flushes because I sweat more and it's harder to feel comfortable when you are overweight.

A bio-psycho-social approach to hot flushes and night sweats

We have seen how biological factors can lead to the development of hot flushes, and, as was the case for the menopause, the experience of symptoms or physical changes can also be influenced by psycho-social and cultural factors. The bio-psycho-social model can, then, be a useful way of thinking about hot flushes and night sweats too (Hunter and Mann 2010) (see Figure 2.2).

Psycho-social factors such as stress have been found to be associated with more problematic hot flushes, as have lifestyle factors such as smoking and low levels of physical activity. Psychological factors can affect our perceptions of hot flushes, such as the situation that we are in, how busy we are, where our attention is focused and the way we think and feel about hot flushes. Day to day, if we are occupied or our attention is focused on something interesting, we are usually less likely to notice a physical symptom. On the other hand, if we closely monitor or focus on a part of the body (known as 'hypervigilance'), research shows that we are likely to notice sensations that we would not normally be aware of. Not surprisingly, sensations that signify something unpleasant or threatening are likely to attract more of our attention: a physical sensation, for example, could be a sign of illness or a temporary, minor ache or pain. There is also some evidence to suggest that certain mood states, such as feeling depressed or anxious, make us more likely to be aware of

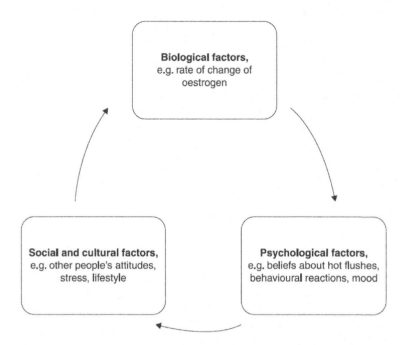

Figure 2.2 A bio-psycho-social approach to hot flushes and night sweats

bodily changes; it is inevitable that when we have been unwell, we are more 'tuned in' to bodily reactions.

As is the case for most symptoms, how we view them and deal with them is likely to make a difference. For example, if we are run down and feeling under the weather, a sudden hot feeling may be interpreted as a sign of being unwell, rather than a hot flush. If a symptom is thought of as common, time-limited or normal, we are unlikely to give it a second thought and are unlikely to visit a doctor. If we worry about what is happening to our body when we have a hot flush or expect that flushes might continue indefinitely, however, we are more likely to feel distressed and seek help. Some women consider a range of explanations when they first have hot flushes before they realize that it may be the menopause.

> When I was 46, I thought that I had a temperature and was having the flu and it wasn't until it continued and I talked to a couple of friends that I realized what it was.

> I was having palpitations at night when I woke up. I was hot and bothered and to be honest, I thought I was having a

heart attack. I woke my husband up in a panic. Eventually I went to the doctor and she said it was the menopause.

Emotional responses and thoughts about hot flushes and menopause highlight the importance of a bio-psycho-social approach when managing menopause and highlight how a talking therapy that looks at thoughts (cognitions), emotions and behaviours may play a role. Anxious thoughts about menopause and hot flushes can result in embarrassment and feelings of being out of control, all of which can make it harder to manage hot flushes and night sweats when they occur. Indeed, several studies have found that these thoughts and reactions about hot flushes are quite common (Hunter and Liao 1995; Rendall *et al*. 2008; Reynolds 2000). It is the uncontrollable and socially embarrassing aspects of hot flushes, as well as the impact of night sweats on sleep, that women find most bothersome and distressing. For example, if we think, 'These flushes are going to go on forever', 'Everyone in the office will think I'm behaving oddly' or 'I'll never get a decent night's sleep again', we are then more likely to experience negative emotional responses alongside the hot flush, which, over time, can make menopause an increasingly distressing experience.

In one study, women who were more distressed in general tended to have more extreme reactions to the physical sensations of flushing as well as more negative, shame-filled attitudes towards themselves, including feeling that they were 'over the hill' or 'not attractive' (Reynolds 1999, 2000). Note that these women did not report such feelings about their bodies or themselves at other times – the thoughts were present mainly when they were experiencing the hot flushes. In contrast, women with low distress reported using encouraging self-talk and other positive strategies during flushing. In these studies, 'catastrophic' thoughts about being out of control, such as 'I cannot possibly concentrate', 'It is terrible and I feel that it is never going to get any better', 'It is awful and I feel that it overwhelms me' and 'I feel like a different person' were associated with greater distress during hot flushes. As you might expect, feeling 'unattractive' or 'useless' during hot flushes also had a negative effect on women's self-esteem.

Interestingly, situations or context can also make a difference. Women generally describe more embarrassment at work when working with men and younger people whom they worry will make negative judgements about them, while working with female colleagues and being able to make a joke about hot flushes can be helpful (Hunter and Liao 1995; Rendall *et al*. 2008; Hunter *et al*. 2009b). These studies together provide evidence that negative appraisals of hot flushes can result in higher levels of distress.

> Having hot flushes makes me feel as if people will know my age and think 'oh, she's menopausal', and think I'm old and past it. . . . I know that sounds weird but I must be thinking that underneath otherwise I wouldn't feel so uncomfortable around people.

In addition, women who have overly negative views and expectations about menopause in general may be more likely to have hot flushes that are distressing (Rendall *et al*. 2008). In Chapter 1, we described how women's expectations of menopause may be influenced by historical ideas about this transition phase in life, which emphasized a very negative view of it being associated with 'ageing and decline' (Hunter and O'Dea 1997, 2001). More negative attitudes to menopause have been found to be associated with more negative beliefs about hot flushes and, in turn, more distressing symptoms (Rendall *et al*. 2008); it is as if, perhaps unconsciously, we are responding with embarrassment or shame to what is actually a normal (if uncomfortable) physical experience as part of a normal life stage.

Most women use a number of practical strategies to alleviate discomfort and to cool down, including the removal of layers of clothing, fanning themselves, attempting to relax and avoiding situations in which they feel uncomfortable (Hunter *et al*. 2011). We will be exploring these beliefs and coping reactions further in the self-help guide, looking at how they interact and helping you to consider what you can put into place to reduce the impact of hot flushes on daily life.

Hot flushes at work

More women are now working during the menopause and some well into their 50s and 60s; for example, in the UK there are over 3.5 million women in employment between the ages of 50 and 65 (Office for National Statistics 2013). There is currently a lot of interest in improving the health and well-being of working women and retaining and increasing the numbers of experienced older women in the workplace.

The menopause at work has become a 'hot topic'! Recent research suggests that many women find menopausal symptoms more difficult to deal with at work, partly due to aspects of the work environment (Griffiths and Hunter 2015). For example, work stress, wearing uniforms, inability to regulate temperature and, importantly, working in a culture where women feel that they have to hide symptoms or their menopause for fear of ridicule and/or lack of understanding can make the situation worse. As well as hot flushes, some women report that tiredness, memory/concentration and loss of confidence are problematic at work. Women are generally reluctant to disclose their menopause status, even if they want to, particularly at work, where embarrassment is common, and self-control is highly valued, particularly during formal meetings, when working with men and/or younger adults or in hot environments.

Some women are worried that their work performance may be affected by menopause. We asked 216 working women aged 45 to 60 to rate their performance as well as other aspects of work, such as work stress, and found that going through the menopause as such was not associated with any work outcomes; instead, self-rated work performance was associated with aspects of the work environment, such as role clarity and work stress. However, women with problematic hot flushes and night sweats were more likely to be considering stopping work (Hardy *et al.* 2018b). So it is important not to expect to have problems at work because you are going through the menopause, but important to find ways to manage troublesome symptoms if they are making you feel that you need to leave work in order to find relief.

We carried out a study (Hardy *et al.* 2017) asking women how they wanted to be treated at work, and this is a summary of their messages to managers and colleagues:

- Be aware that menopause is a normal process, not an affliction, that varies between women; avoid a 'one-size-fits-all' approach.
  'Don't make assumptions based on prejudices, on generalizations or on experiences of other individuals'.
  'Be aware that women might have difficulty being in warm/hot office environments at such times'.
- Listen, be respectful, take seriously, offer privacy; don't joke, patronize, criticize or view women as less competent.
- Have supportive policies for staff training and awareness.

*'Managers should be provided with training and equipped
with skills to discuss personal issues with staff'.*

These points are consistent with those included in recent guidance for employers (Griffiths and Hunter 2015). Based on these
recommendations, we carried out a three-year study to (i) develop
and test a brief online training for managers and (ii) find out if
CBT for menopausal symptoms was effective in the workplace – a
non-clinical setting. We found that the training improved managers' knowledge and attitudes to menopause and their confidence
in talking about it sensitively should the need arise (Hardy *et al.*
2019). The results of the CBT for working women were also very
positive (Hardy *et al.* 2018a) and are described on pages 51–52.

Hot flushes following breast cancer treatment

Hot flushes are common among women who have been diagnosed with, and treated for, breast cancer. Breast cancer is the
most common form of this disease diagnosed in women in the
UK (Office for National Statistics 2010), but with better detec-
tion and treatments, more women are living for longer after
treatment. However, some treatments for breast cancer have
additional side effects, which can include hot flushes, night
sweats and sleep problems (Fenlon *et al.* 2009). They affect
women who become menopausal following chemotherapy and
also women who are having endocrine or hormone treatment
for breast cancer, such as tamoxifen or aromatase inhibitors,
such Arimidex, because these hormone therapies reduce oestrogen levels. About 65 per cent of breast cancers are oestrogen
receptor positive, i.e. they need oestrogen to grow (Ellis 2007).
So hormonal therapies for breast cancer are used to block the
production of oestrogen or limit its ability to reach the tumour
cells that need it to grow. Hot flushes and night sweats are
often more severe amongst breast cancer survivors due to the
rapid reduction in oestrogen levels and can be associated with
sleep problems and reduced health-related quality of life (Carpenter *et al.* 2002; Hunter *et al.* 2004; Gupta *et al.* 2006b).

Most women who develop breast cancer have already gone
through the menopause – the risk of developing breast cancer
increases with age – and they may well have been experiencing
menopausal symptoms when their cancer was first discovered.
Women who have previously been taking HRT for hot flushes may
be advised to stop the treatment when breast cancer is diagnosed,
because oestrogen can increase the risk of the cancer's recurrence.

For premenopausal breast cancer sufferers, treatment with chemotherapy or tamoxifen can induce or increase the severity of menopausal symptoms. The abrupt onset of menopausal symptoms can be particularly distressing for younger women because of concerns about fertility; women also have to deal with the psychological and physical impact of being 'menopausal' well before they would have expected to undergo that transition.

Women undergoing treatment for gynaecological cancers can also experience menopausal symptoms following medical intervention. They may have had their ovaries removed, for example, which causes rapid reduction in oestrogen levels. And, as mentioned in the previous chapter, prostate cancer treatment can result in hot flushes and night sweats for men too. These symptoms occur in response to the lowering of testosterone caused by the treatments. It is estimated that somewhere between 34 and 80 per cent of prostate cancer patients report hot flushes following androgen deprivation treatment. However, hot flushes are less well researched for men than for female breast cancer sufferers.

Studies of women's experience of hot flushes following breast cancer (Fenlon *et al.* 2009; Hunter *et al.* 2009) highlight the distress associated with feeling that their bodies are out of control, a longing to feel 'normal' again after a period of tiring treatments and at a time when there is less contact with oncology services. Other symptoms include fatigue, concerns about body image, depression and anxiety. Night sweats can affect sleep, resulting in fatigue; similarly, feeling tired or depressed can affect a woman's ability to cope with hot flushes. As noted earlier, being rendered suddenly menopausal can be particularly difficult for younger women facing the loss or impairment of fertility as well as dealing with changes in body image. The CBT approach for hot flushes in the self-help guide (see Chapters 4–7) is effective for women who have had breast cancer too (Mann *et al.* 2012; Atema *et al.* 2019) and has been found to help men to manage these symptoms following prostate cancer treatments (Stefanopoulou *et al.* 2015). Other specific needs can be addressed by cancer psychological support services, primary care counselling services or cancer charities (see Resources, pages 168–169).

What can help?

Hormone treatments for hot flushes

HRT is an effective treatment for hot flushes in otherwise healthy women (Archer *et al.* 2011; NICE 2015b) and includes both oestrogen therapy and combined oestrogen and progestogen therapy. 'Progestogen' refers to both progesterone and progestin; progestogens cause a monthly menstrual bleed and are prescribed in order to prevent cancer of the womb. (Women who have had a hysterectomy do not need to add the progesterone to oestrogen.) HRT can be used in a variety of forms, from pills to skin patches and creams. HRT has been prescribed to combat hot flushes and night sweats and for vaginal dryness and has also been recommended for the prevention of osteoporosis. HRT can help to prevent bone loss and therefore reduces the risk of osteoporosis if used in the early postmenopause, but the effects lessen when the treatment is stopped. Menopausal symptoms can also recur when HRT is stopped, but gradually reducing HRT may lessen the recurrence of symptoms (NICE 2015b).

As mentioned in the Introduction, since 2002 there has been concern about the long-term safety of HRT following the publication of observational studies and clinical trials (Rossouw et al. 2002; Manson et al. 2003; Beral 2003) associating HRT use with increased risks of breast cancer, thrombosis and stroke. Following publication of these trials, HRT use declined in the UK between 2002 and 2005 from approximately 30 to 10 per cent (Menon et al. 2007); a similar sustained reduction to low levels has been identified in a large US study of over 10,000 women. The study found that in 2009 and 2010, less than 5 per cent of postmenopausal women over the age of 40 were using either HRT (oestrogen alone or oestrogen and progestin), compared to about 22 per cent in 1999 and 2000 (Sprague et al. 2012).

NICE guidance has reviewed the more recent evidence, taking into account criticisms of the methods used in some of the studies. For example, the US Women's Health Initiative study has been criticized because it included 50- to 70-year-old women with an average age of 63. In summary, the NICE guidance (2015b) recommends that for women with menopausal symptoms, the risks of HRT, such as breast cancer, deep vein thrombosis and stroke, are relatively small and usually outweighed by the benefits (www.nice.org.uk/guidance/NG23; go to Information for the public for short summaries).

A central theme of the guidance is the need to inform women of the risks and benefits of HRT so that they can make appropriate treatment choices; for a good summary of pros and cons, see Abernethy (2018) and/or Women's Health Concern Fact

Sheet on HRT pros and cons (www.womens-health-concern. org/wp-content/uploads/2015/02/WHC-FACTSHEET-HRT-Ben efitsRisks-NOV17.pdf). There are several different forms of HRT, so if you are using it and have any concerns, do discuss these with your doctor. Survivors of breast cancer and some gynaecological cancers are usually advised to avoid oestrogen (and HRT) for fear of stimulating tumour growth (Verheul *et al.* 2000). It is also important to remember that women who have early menopause are advised to continue with HRT up until the natural age of menopause, i.e. 50 years (Panay and Fenton 2008). Concerns about side effects and long-term safety of HT have contributed to an increased interest in non-hormonal treatments, informed choices for women and self-management approaches.

Non-hormonal treatments for hot flushes

Non-hormonal medical treatments, such as selective serotonin and noradrenaline reuptake inhibitors (SSRIs and SNRIs, which are mainly used as antidepressants), clonidine (an antihypertensive medication) and gabapentin (an anticonvulsant) have been found to be moderately effective in the treatment of hot flushes (NAMS 2015; Hickey *et al.* 2017). However, side effects are reported, including dizziness, fatigue, mouth dryness, decreased appetite, nausea and constipation, which might limit their use for some women. If you are taking tamoxifen to reduce breast cancer risk, you should avoid the SSRIs fluoxetine and paroxetine since these can reduce the effectiveness of the tamoxifen. Of the medications mentioned here, clonidine is the only licensed non-hormonal medicine for the treatment of menopausal symptoms in the UK, which means that there is no information included for you in the information sheets of the other treatments.

Complementary therapies, such as vitamins, herbal remedies and reflexology, are popular, but recent reviews of the research suggest that there is insufficient evidence to be confident about their effectiveness overall (Borrelli and Ernst 2010; Franco *et al.* 2016; Pitkin 2012; NICE 2015b; NAMS 2015). NICE (2015b) concludes that while there is mixed evidence, black cohosh (used in small doses of 40 mg) and isoflavones (e.g. soy-based products called phytoestrogens that are plant-derived substances that mimic oestrogen in their action) may help hot flushes and night sweats. Some interactions with other medicines have been reported, and black cohosh should not be used if you have had liver damage or if you have had breast cancer; similarly, isoflavones are not usually recommended for women who have had breast cancer (Woyka 2017).

There are mixed results, but also some positive findings, for acupuncture (Befus *et al.* 2018). Yoga, mindfulness and exercise have been found to offer general benefits, for example to sleep and well-being, rather than having specific impacts on hot flushes and night sweats (NAMS 2015; Hickey *et al.* 2017).

Therefore, there is a need for safe and effective non-hormonal treatments that are free from side effects to help both well women and breast cancer survivors manage these symptoms. Women going through the menopause often prefer non-medical treatments unless their symptoms are severe, in which case some want a rapid and effective medical treatment. In a survey of breast cancer patients (Hunter *et al.* 2004), we found that women had rarely used treatments for menopausal symptoms in the past but were keen to find an effective solution for their hot flushes. When asked, they expressed preferences for non-hormonal treatments, with over 60 per cent preferring complementary therapies or self-management interventions.

Cognitive behavioural approaches for hot flushes

Over the past 30 years we have developed a CBT intervention specifically for menopausal symptoms, which includes relaxation; calm, paced breathing; and cognitive behavioural therapy (Hunter and Liao 1996; Hunter 2003). It is based on years of research demonstrating the significant impact that psycho-social factors can have on women's experience of menopause. Therefore, this CBT approach was developed to help women to examine attitudes and beliefs about menopause, hot flushes and night sweats (i.e., assumptions and beliefs about menopause and cognitive appraisal of hot flushes and night sweats), and behavioural reactions to them. It provides evidence-based information and exploration of attributions and social meanings and cognitive behavioural strategies to deal with hot flushes, night sweats, and broader lifestyle issues that play a role in menopausal symptoms, including stress and sleep. The aim of CBT when applied to menopause is to help you identify unhelpful or overly negative beliefs and behaviours in relation to menopause and menopausal symptoms to enable you to develop self-supportive and proactive management strategies. We have trialled the treatment in a range of studies which have demonstrated CBT to have a range of benefits that facilitate improved coping. These are detailed later in the text. CBT is described in more detail in the next chapter. The self-help guide we developed as part of the research – CBT for hot flushes and night sweats (Chapters 4–7) – is the interactive four-session intervention tested in our research trials.

We evaluated the treatment in different formats (one-to-one with a psychologist, in groups of six to eight women and as a self-help booklet and online) by comparing these forms of CBT with no treatment or usual care respectively.

We carried out two initial randomised controlled trials (the gold standard method of testing whether a treatment works) of CBT, which have recently been completed:

1 MENOS 1 – for women who have hot flushes following breast cancer treatment; and
2 MENOS 2 – for well women going through the menopause transition.

The studies included over 200 women who had frequent and troublesome hot flushes and night sweats, and the results were positive and consistent across the trials. Results of both trials (Ayers *et al.* 2012; Mann *et al.* 2012) showed that these CBT interventions are effective in reducing the impact, or problem rating, of hot flushes and night sweats and have additional benefits to mood and quality of life. We also found that there were small but significant improvements in memory and concentration for those women who had had CBT compared with those who had not. This was the case in both trials, i.e. for well women going through the menopause transition (Ayers *et al.* 2012) and for those who had hot flushes following treatment for breast cancer (Mann *et al.* 2012). These findings support the existing evidence that stress and mood, as well as hot flushes and night sweats, are associated with subjective reports of memory problems.

We compared both group and self-help formats of the CBT in MENOS 2 and found that both were equally effective in reducing problematic hot flushes and night sweats. Women who used the self-help guide had significant improvements in menopausal symptoms (hot flushes and night sweats) six weeks and six months afterwards, compared with a control group who did not read the self-help guide. The self-help guide, used over a four-week period, was found to be as effective as four two-hour weekly sessions of group CBT. As a result of the treatment, over 70 per cent of the women who entered the study with problematic symptoms obtained clinically significant improvements that were maintained at the six month follow-up; their symptoms were rendered less bothersome and the frequency of night sweats significantly reduced.

Further analyses of MENOS 1 and 2 suggest that CBT appears to work by changing women's perceptions, attitudes and beliefs (the cognitive part of CBT) about menopause and menopausal symptoms and increasing behavioural strategies, such as calm breathing (Chilcot *et al*. 2014; Norton *et al*. 2014). In-depth interviews with participants at the end of MENOS 1 and 2 trials were conducted to find out what women thought about the treatment. Women reported increased confidence and ability to cope with hot flushes and night sweats; key factors mentioned were acceptance and a restored sense of control (experienced on a number of different levels and often facilitated by calm breathing). Many women noticed a change in their experience of hot flushes once they started to implement the strategies outlined; for example, they may have had hot flushes but did not notice them. Perhaps reflecting the skills learned, the beneficial effects of the treatment, in some cases, extended beyond management of menopausal symptoms. Some women also found the group context helpful in terms of normalizing their experiences, motivating them in homework tasks and providing support (Balabanovic *et al*. 2012, 2013).

We are collaborating with a Dutch research team who have published the results of two CBT trials:

1 Comparing the same CBT with physical exercise for women who had hot flushes following breast cancer treatment. These women were all premenopausal, i.e. younger women, when breast cancer was diagnosed (Duijts *et al*. 2012). The results of this study were similar to those of our MENOS 1 and MENOS 2 trials, showing significant improvements with CBT. CBT had more impact on how troublesome hot flushes were rated than did no treatment or physical activity alone.
2 An online version of the self-help CBT was developed and modified for breast cancer patients and found to be effective both with and without health professional guidance by telephone or email (Atema *et al*. 2019). Again, the treatment had additional impact on quality of life.

Our most recent study aimed to improve the working lives for working women with troublesome menopausal symptoms from eight UK organisations (Hardy *et al*. 2018a). Sixty women were given the self-help CBT book for hot flushes and night sweats, symptoms that can be difficult to manage in work contexts due to physical discomfort, social embarrassment, sleep disturbance and aspects of the work environment. Six weeks later the women rated their menopausal symptoms as significantly less problematic, reported improvements in sleep quality and viewed menopause as more controllable, compared to a control group of 64 women who did not receive the CBT. The treated women also rated their work and social adjustment as improved, and they felt that menopausal symptoms interfered less with their working lives.

CBT for menopausal symptoms has been shown to be helpful for women who have these symptoms plus depression (Green *et al.* 2019) and is being offered in community settings with minority ethnic groups (for example, Bellott *et al.* 2018) and is available in some clinical settings in the UK both in group and self-help formats. We have published a manual for trained health professionals to run CBT groups for women with troublesome menopausal symptoms (Hunter and Smith 2015), and there is now an annual training course for health professionals run by Melanie Smith and Janet Balabanovic, organised by the British Menopause Society (see BMS website in Resources). The self-help CBT was presented as part of a recent BBC TV programme hosted by Mariella Frostrup, 'The Truth about Menopause' – the five women who took part found that the CBT was very helpful reporting significant improvements in symptoms. One participant described the intervention as 'life changing'. Interestingly, the women formed a WhatsApp group and encouraged each other during the four weeks of treatment.

In summary, hot flushes and night sweats are common but can disrupt everyday life and affect sleep. Although they are not dangerous, they can make it hard to get the most out of life, and consequently they can have a detrimental impact on our mood and well-being. They are physiological reactions to lowering levels of oestrogen during the menopause or can be a consequence of medical or surgical treatments. However, it is important to remember that they are not signs of disease. It is difficult to predict who will have hot flushes, so it makes sense for all women to adopt a healthy lifestyle as far as possible in order to reduce some of the possible risk factors: taking steps to stop smoking, manage weight during the menopause and engage in some physical activity can only ever be positive.

There is a range of treatments available that have varied levels of effectiveness. There is substantial evidence, with studies including over 1,000 women, that the CBT approach featured in this book is effective in reducing the impact of hot flushes and that it was acceptable to women who took part in our studies. They reported both specific improvements in hot flushes and night sweats but as an additional benefit, also learned some general skills that they could apply to a range of situations. In the next chapter, CBT is explained in more detail, with examples of its application to psychological and physical conditions.

3

A cognitive behavioural approach

What is cognitive behavioural therapy?

We have described the evidence showing that CBT can reduce the impact hot flushes have on women's day-to-day lives. It can also improve general well-being. So you may be left wondering how a psychological or 'talking' therapy can help you deal with hot flushes, which are physical symptoms. Furthermore, you may be asking if we are suggesting that there is a psychological cause for hot flushes and night sweats and that simply talking about them is enough to stop or get rid of them. This is not the case. Although CBT comes under the umbrella term of 'talking therapies', it does not involve simply talking about a health issue; instead, CBT broadens what is essentially a biomedical approach to a bio-psycho-social approach.

CBT for physical health problems

Often, and not surprisingly, people tend to think that offering a 'psychological' treatment for a physical symptom means that the physical symptom is caused by psychological factors. They fear that it is 'all in their head' or that they are 'going mad' in some way. We are brought up to view the mind and body as separate entities, but in fact health conditions affect us at all levels, and psychological, social and biological factors can influence our experience of illnesses.

For example, being diagnosed with a long-term (chronic) health condition can have a profound impact on a person's beliefs about themselves, their place in the world and their future (Taylor 2005; White 2001). People suddenly become aware of their own mortality, something that they may not have considered before, especially when the condition that they are diagnosed with happens only to 'other people'. They can easily feel vulnerable because they might always have thought themselves to be 'strong and healthy' prior to the diagnosis. Quite understandably, their confidence is rocked, and they start to worry about the future. The unpredictability of symptoms for some health conditions, as well as the severity of symptoms, can impact upon lifestyle including hobbies, as well as ability to work and to fulfil important roles. The stress arising from these changes can then influence people's experience of their illness, setting up a vicious cycle. Consequently, people with long-term health conditions are at increased risk of experiencing depression or anxiety (White 2001), which can have a negative impact on long-term health.

Diabetes offers us a good example of how biological factors (the health condition) and psycho-social factors interact. Research demonstrates that factors such as daily stress, beliefs and understanding of the illness and medication, as well as mood, can all have an impact on how well somebody manages their blood sugar levels (Nicolucci *et al.* 2013), which is the primary focus of medical management. Furthermore, psycho-social interventions such as CBT, which target these issues, have been shown to improve long-term glucose control, physical health outcomes and quality of life (Harkness *et al.* 2010) and are an integral part of NHS guidelines for the management of diabetes (NICE 2015a). There is evidence to show that CBT can be a useful tool in the management of a broad range of health conditions, such as chronic pain (Morley *et al.* 1999), insomnia (Espie 2010), irritable bowel syndrome (McCrone *et al.* 2008) and chronic fatigue (Chalder 1995).

Because of this, psychologists often work with doctors, nurses and other health professionals as part of multidisciplinary teams. Psychologists may work with patients individually or in groups to help them to understand and adjust to health conditions with the aim of reducing the negative impact of the illness and improving quality of life. In this context CBT often involves relaxation and stress management, increasing meaningful activities (which might include exercise as well as having a structure to the day with a range of activities) and practical problem-solving, as well as understanding and addressing negative emotions. CBT also aims to help people improve their confidence or self-efficacy in relation to their health condition (their view of their ability to deal with it), which can have a positive impact on their mood and quality of life.

CBT and menopause symptoms

In the previous chapter, we reviewed some of the research highlighting how broader psycho-social factors such as beliefs, general stress and emotions can all interact. CBT for menopause symptoms aims to draw all this research together and identify the things that have been shown to help women to cope with symptoms and reduce their impact on quality of life. The CBT workbook therefore aims to help you look at how menopause symptoms interact with other areas that you are able to influence such as stress, lifestyle, thinking and behaviour and help you apply changes that research shows can have a positive impact on menopause symptoms.

Changing thinking and behaviour

Behaviour change, such as stopping smoking, going on a diet or doing more exercise, can be really challenging and is actually a complex process involving a range of factors (Prochaska and Velicer 1997). Why is this relevant to menopausal symptoms? Because, essentially the self-help section of the book is focused on helping you to change aspects of your current situation such as your coping responses (the 'psycho' of the bio-psycho-social) and change how you deal with stressors (the 'social' of the bio-psycho-social) to reduce the impact of menopause symptoms on your quality of life.

Behaviour change has been found to take place over five stages:

1 pre-contemplation (not ready to change);
2 contemplation (getting ready to change);
3 preparation (ready to change);
4 action; and
5 maintenance.

Buying this book shows you have started to think about what you can do to help yourself to manage menopausal symptoms (contemplation). Reading through the self-help guide and learning more about the interaction between menopausal symptoms and psycho-social influences would come under the 'preparation' stage, and putting strategies into practice shows that you have moved into the 'action' stage. The initial action and maintenance stages tend to be the trickiest bits, as it is often during these stages that you have to think about adapting strategies to your specific situation or deal with barriers that may get in the way of change. The self-help guide is designed to help you to anticipate potential barriers and learn from these when they happen. Awareness of these stages of change has helped people to improve the way they manage stress, lose weight, stop smoking and change behaviour.

The influence of thoughts and feelings on behaviour

So before we start the self-help guide, it can be helpful to know a bit more about CBT. Cognitive behavioural therapy literally means thinking about (cognitive) and doing (behaviour) things differently. In the context of menopause, the cognitive part refers to all of the thinking processes that take place when you notice and experience a symptom, such as hot flushes or insomnia, or how you look at broader influences such as stress; the behaviour part is what you do in response to a hot flush, insomnia or stress. Reading through the research in the previous chapter and working through the self-help book will help you to increase your knowledge and understanding of hot flushes and menopause more generally, but it is proactively applying this knowledge in real-life situations (by using the self-help guide to change thinking and behaviour) that will make the difference.

CBT revolutionised our understanding of psychological distress and how we cope with challenging situations. It was initially developed in the 1960s and 70s by an American psychiatrist, Aaron Beck, who noticed that distress in his anxious and depressed patients was preceded by specific patterns of thinking (Beck 1976). Before this time, therapeutic approaches focused mainly on behaviour change through reinforcement (rewarding certain behaviours) or psychoanalytic approaches, which focused on patterns of interaction in past and current relationships. Beck added the 'cognitive' or thinking part to behaviour therapy, and cognitive behavioural therapy was born. CBT offered a pragmatic and practical approach to emotional problems, such as anxiety and depression, and over the past few decades CBT has been applied to a range of mental health and physical health problems with impressive results. People with physical health issues including back pain, chronic fatigue and cancer have responded well to CBT (Gatchel and Rollings 2008; Chambers et al. 2006; Moorey et al. 1994). CBT has led to improvements in coping strategies and a reduction in the emotional distress that can arise when living with chronic health conditions (Sage et al. 2008). Consequently, it often offers broader benefits to patients in terms of ability to enjoy and cope with daily life.

CBT is a structured and time-limited intervention (Middleton *et al*. 2005). This is quite different from common stereotypes of talking therapies, which may conjure up images of a person lying on a couch talking about their childhood. Instead, CBT focuses on the 'here and now', with therapists and patients working together to identify and address factors contributing to their current emotional well-being. Patients take an active role in therapy and over time become their own 'expert' in understanding and managing their psychological well-being, working towards meaningful goals. Outside of sessions, patients complete homework tasks, in which they apply information and strategies identified within sessions. Initially, homework often involves monitoring thinking, feelings and behaviours in situations they find difficult. This information gathering can help them to change unhelpful patterns and build adaptive coping skills.

The central premise of CBT is that our perspective within situations (our thinking) influences how we feel and what we do (our behaviour) in that situation. Evaluating a situation objectively by considering all factors that contribute to it can lead to a reduction in psychological distress within challenging situations and subsequently increases the likelihood of responding in a more helpful way.

To demonstrate these links, a CBT approach breaks down these 'trigger' situations into separate components or systems: details about the situation that leads to emotional distress, thinking patterns within that situation, common emotional responses, behaviours and physiological responses. It seeks to understand how these different components interact with each other, setting up a vicious cycle. Figure 3.1 illustrates how these components can link up and reinforce each other. The diagram links the components up in a 'hot cross bun' model, which helps us understand how the different components lead to and reinforce other parts of the system (Padesky and Mooney 1990).

We will use a situation that many of us may identify with, such as breaking a healthy eating plan or diet. Let's see how the contrasting thinking patterns of two individuals, both of whom are in the 'action' stage of behaviour change, may have quite different influences on how they feel and cope within the same situation, which then has longer-term implications for how quickly they get back to healthy eating.

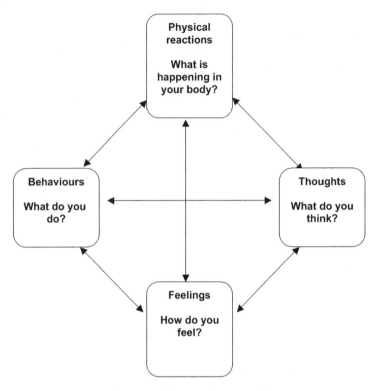

Figure 3.1 Cognitive behavioural 'hot cross bun' model

Emma

Thoughts: I've blown my diet. I'll never lose weight. I have no willpower.

Feelings: Fed-up, hopeless, disappointed with self.

Behaviour: Gives up on diet and resumes less healthy eating/bingeing patterns.

Physical reactions: Tension, gains weight in the long term.

Debby

Thoughts: Oh well, I can carry on with it later/tomorrow. One little slip won't make a difference – I've been doing very well until now.

Feelings: Optimistic.

Behaviour: Resumes diet at next meal or next day.

Physical reactions: None, loses weight in long term.

From these examples, you can see how the two different thinking responses, can lead to very different emotional, behavioural and physical consequences. Emma is self-critical and interprets the event as 'total failure' on her part, rather than a blip in an otherwise successful plan. She then feels really disappointed and is hard on herself, leading her to give up. In the long term, this may lead her to regain any weight she has lost, or it may take her longer to get back into the planning and action stage of her healthy eating plan, which will reinforce her initial negative thinking. Effectively, a 'vicious cycle' has been set up, which Emma may find difficult to step out of because of how the different responses feed into and reinforce each other.

In contrast, Debby responds in a calmer and more self-supportive manner. She acknowledges the 'hiccup', but it is viewed as a blip, and instead she focuses on what she has achieved. This means that intense negative emotions are avoided, and in the long run she is more likely to get back into the 'action' stage and maintain change to achieve her goal.

The role of thoughts

One of the fundamental principles of CBT is that thoughts are not necessarily facts but one perspective on a given situation. Thoughts play a pivotal role in our emotions and behaviour, and yet we are not always fully aware of them. Thoughts are automatic and rapid, forming a running commentary that may trigger other thoughts or memories. We can be engaged in an activity or situation, such as work or a social event, and at the same time be thinking about something completely different. When people practise meditation or relaxation, they suddenly become aware of the relentless nature of thinking; try spending a minute not thinking about anything and see what happens – it is highly unlikely that your mind will empty and remain clear. In fact, within a matter of seconds, your attention will probably drift on to what you need to do later today, what you did last week or when you're going on your next holiday. And each time you try to refocus your thoughts, they start off again on another tangent. Our minds are naturally very busy.

One of the main characteristics of thinking that Beck noticed when people experienced emotional distress was that they tended to be susceptible to common thinking biases. People who feel depressed tend to be overly negative in their evaluation of themselves (e.g. 'I'm completely useless'), their situation (e.g. 'It's hopeless; there's nothing I can do') or what the future may hold (e.g. 'It will never get any better'). When we experience anxiety (or stress), we tend to interpret situations by focusing on potential threats and danger within the situation (Beck 1976). As well as emotional consequences, these thinking patterns typically lead to behaviours that reinforce initial thinking patterns: social withdrawal by depressed people or avoidance of a feared situation for people prone to anxiety. This can then set up a vicious cycle that can keep low mood or anxiety going, because the thinking patterns remain unchallenged. For example, because anxious people actively avoid certain situations, they may not give themselves the opportunity to find out that the feared situations are safe.

CBT aims to help people to understand and be more aware of their thinking when they experience negative emotional reactions. Over time, CBT provides patients with the tools to help them question these responses and to come up with more helpful alternatives that reduce emotional distress. This does not mean simply substituting a negative perspective for 'positive thinking' that you don't really believe, but systematically 'examining' thoughts by taking a step back, considering the evidence and looking at the situation from a different and more constructive perspective.

We are not saying that all negative emotions just need 'positive thinking' or that they are inappropriate. When we experience a major disappointment or a loss, such as bereavement, the attendant, powerful emotions of grief are normal and functional, in that they help us come to terms with our loss and, over time, adjust to it. Furthermore, emotions serve a useful function that helps to identify threats, motivates us to work towards goals and encourages us to rest and recuperate (Gilbert 2009). CBT has an important role to play for anyone experiencing distress or negative feelings frequently in response to everyday life or arising from living with a long-term health condition, as these negative emotions can start to create their own problems.

Where does thinking come from?

Our thinking is very much influenced by our general or core beliefs about ourselves, about others and about the world. These beliefs develop throughout life starting in childhood and are influenced by our life experiences. If we have positive messages in our formative years and go on to have some positive life experiences as we grow up, we are probably more likely to view ourselves, others and the world in general in a neutral or positive light. These protective self-beliefs can help us to cope when stresses crop up (Blenkiron 2005). There is also evidence that some stress can help people to develop strengths and resilience (Bandura 1995).

In the earlier example, it is likely that Emma has some negative core beliefs about herself in that her self-worth may rest on doing well. She may have high standards that she developed when she was younger (perhaps from being naturally a 'high achiever' and having parents who overvalued achievement), which now influence how she responds to setbacks. For Emma, missing her diet goal is interpreted in a 'black-and-white' way as 'total failure'. Debby, on the other hand, may have experienced encouragement from her parents so that any setbacks she encountered when she was younger may have been met with encouragement – 'You did your best; try again next time'. Debby will have internalised this approach, so she is naturally more self-supportive as an adult when encountering difficulties. For Emma to successfully maintain her weight-loss programme, it is likely that she will also need to be aware of and address her thinking patterns, where they may have arisen from and how they link into her responses to setbacks in her diet.

CBT for common mental health problems

In the UK, recognition of CBT's effectiveness is demonstrated by its inclusion in the National Institute for Health and Clinical Excellence (NICE) guidelines for several health issues (name changed from Clinical to Care Excellence in 2013). The NICE guidelines are essentially clinical parameters for good practice for both mental and physical health issues based on the best available evidence. This has, in turn, led to the development and implementation of the Improving Access to Psychological Therapies (IAPT) programme within the National Health Service (NHS) (Department of Health 2008). IAPT was developed to deliver low- and high-intensity CBT interventions for people with mild or moderate-to-severe depression and anxiety, in addition to medication or as a stand-alone therapy. The programme was initially aimed at people of working age, but is now available to all adults and, increasingly, to people with health problems and long-term conditions (NHS England 2016).

CBT for depression

CBT is currently one of the principal recommended treatments for depression in the UK today (National Institute for Health and

Clinical Excellence 2009). A good deal of research has been done on the effectiveness of CBT for depression in clinical settings, and it has also featured in research trials over the years. Reviews of these trials tend to indicate that for mild-to-moderate depression, self-help and computerized CBT are helpful (Anderson *et al.* 2005; Høifødt *et al.* 2011), while for moderate-to-severe depression, CBT or a combination of CBT and antidepressants are the best options (Pampallona *et al.* 2004; Whitfield and Williams 2003; NICE 2006). Compared to treating depression with antidepressants alone, CBT results in a lower risk of relapse, i.e. people are less likely to have another bout of depression (Paykel *et al.* 2005).

Early on in CBT treatment, patients are encouraged to re-engage in activities that they previously valued and enjoyed but which they have withdrawn from since becoming depressed. This 'behavioural activation' and developing a structure to the day can help to initially lift mood and generally precedes work on thinking patterns. However, the overall aims of CBT are led by the patient, in order to be consistent with the individual's beliefs and values; an important part of the therapy is to enable people to value their own qualities, strengths and competencies (Beck *et al.* 1979). Because CBT involves learning skills for life in terms of managing distress by changing thinking and behaviour, it is particularly useful in maintaining improvements in mood. It also helps people to avoid relapses by enabling them to spot the early signs of stress or low mood and to then implement the relevant CBT strategies.

For example, when asked about work, Jenny says, 'I just do what I'm asked to do and even then, I'm not very good at it – no one appreciates what I do anyway'. However, when the details of her day-to-day work and the feedback that she had received from her boss and colleagues were explored in session, she was able to recall positive comments from her appraisal and how she consistently meets deadlines at work. It is easy not to remember or to notice the good things when we are feeling low.

Box 3.1 What are the symptoms of depression?

- Loss of interest in things that you previously enjoyed.
- Feeling down, depressed or hopeless.
- Feeling irritable and restless or also feeling 'slowed down'.

- Negative thoughts and feelings about yourself, e.g. feeling unloved or that you are a failure.
- Difficulty with concentration, for example, reading or watching TV.
- Sleep disturbance, such as difficulty falling asleep or staying asleep or sleeping too much.
- Poor appetite or eating too much.
- Suicidal thoughts.

Box 3.2 What can help?

- Regular exercise can help to relieve depression. NICE guidelines have recommended structured, supervised exercise programmes, three times a week (45 minutes to one hour) over 10 to 14 weeks, as a treatment for mild-to-moderate depression (National Institute for Health and Clinical Excellence 2009). There are also benefits for people with moderate-to-severe depression (Rimer *et al*. 2012).
- Psychological treatments for depression, particularly CBT, have been recommended in the UK NICE guidelines (National Institute for Health and Clinical Excellence 2009) and are provided in the UK on the NHS.
- Antidepressant medication is an effective and commonly used treatment for moderate-to-severe depression, although some people experience side effects (Agency for Health Research and Quality (AHRQ) 2012).
- If you think that you might be or are suffering from depression, then do discuss this with your doctor, who can offer you the appropriate treatment.

CBT for anxiety

Detailed reviews of all available research (meta-analyses) demonstrate that CBT is consistently effective in treating anxiety and is considered to be the gold standard in psychological treatments for anxiety disorders (Hofmann and Smits 2008; Otte 2011). As for depression, CBT is often considered preferable to taking medication over the long term as it offers people an understanding of how thoughts and behaviours maintain anxiety and reduces the risk of relapse.

The CBT model of anxiety disorders identifies 'anxious thinking', such as predicting the worst possible outcomes in situations or viewing these situations as unnecessarily threatening, as contributing to and maintaining anxiety. For people with social anxiety, this can mean assuming that others will judge them negatively in social situations, and, as a result, sufferers are likely to avoid these social occasions (Clark and Wells 1995). People with panic disorder (commonly known as agoraphobia) tend to misinterpret anxiety symptoms in the body as being signs of imminent disaster, such as 'going mad,' fainting or losing control. These anxious thoughts may then trigger a panic attack, which is associated with rapid 'chest breathing', increased heart rate and other physical symptoms (Clark 1986). People with health anxiety (a term that replaced the unhelpful label of hypochondriasis) tend to misinterpret benign or normal physical sensations as signs of serious disease and become overly worried about their health. If health anxiety becomes severe and chronic, some people can end up having too many hospital investigations or even unnecessary (and occasionally damaging) treatments (Warwick and Salkovskis 1990).

Behaviour is also important, as people experiencing these difficulties tend to employ a range of 'safety' behaviours – such as the avoidance of anxiety-provoking situations – that can help them cope with their anxiety in the short term, but which actually keep fuelling anxiety in the long run (Salkovskis 1991). For example, someone with social anxiety might try to conceal symptoms of social embarrassment by not making eye contact with others or hiding in the corner of a room. Paradoxically, these 'safety behaviours' don't help them to overcome their anxiety but can keep it going in the long term. People with panic disorder often deal with anxiety by avoiding situations completely and thinking that they have avoided disaster when their anxiety, although unpleasant, is unlikely to have such catastrophic consequences. People with health anxiety tend to monitor – or become hyper-vigilant of – the symptoms that they fear. They may, for example, repeatedly check their pulse to reassure themselves that their heart is beating normally.

But as you might expect, monitoring symptoms has the opposite effect to that intended, because it can increase awareness of normal bodily experiences. Rather than allay fears, it can cause anxiety to continue or indeed increase.

CBT approaches to treating anxiety educate people about anxiety using a bio-psycho-social approach and help them to examine how anxious thinking tends to overestimate the likelihood of the worst-case scenario happening. In time, the person with anxiety is helped to develop more neutral, realistic responses by 'testing' their thoughts against available evidence and information. They are also given skills to remain in their feared situation, which, over time, aim to help directly challenge their anxious assumptions about the situation and build confidence. Again, we are all anxious sometimes, and it is a normal reaction to certain situations. Anxiety, like pain, has developed because it can be important for survival, but we are referring here to specific ways of interpreting benign and non-dangerous situations and events.

Box 3.3 What are symptoms of anxiety?

Physical reactions give us the energy to fight or run away (the 'fight or flight' response) and can include:

- A racing heart. This takes the blood to where it is most needed: for example, to the arms, legs and lungs. These changes can cause tingling, coldness and numbness.
- Breathing faster. This helps the bloodstream to carry oxygen to the arms and legs but can lead to chest pain and breathlessness. As there is a slight drop in the oxygen being sent to the brain, we may feel dizzy or light headed.
- Sweating. This helps to cool the muscles and stop the body from overheating.
- The digestive system slowing down. This can lead to nausea, 'butterflies' and a dry mouth.
- Becoming more alert. We are focused on looking for danger and, as a result, become less able to concentrate on anything else.

Emotional reactions include:

- Feelings of fear, anxiety and sometimes panic. We worry that something terrible will happen, that we might faint or collapse.
- Commonly recurring negative thoughts. These often focus on the worst possible scenario that could happen ('catastrophizing') and the idea that we won't be able to cope with the consequences.

Behaviours might include:

- Avoiding challenging situations, such as people or places.
- Going to certain places only at certain times or only in the company of someone else.
- Less helpful strategies for dealing with anxiety, including using alcohol or food.

The following strategies can be used to break the vicious cycle of anxious thoughts, emotions and behaviours:

- Practise calm, diaphragmatic breathing, breathing slowly from the stomach. This can help reduce the physical sensations, emotions and intensity of thoughts. We describe this in detail in the self-help guide (see pages 87–88). Yoga, relaxation and meditation can help to reduce the physical reactions.

- At times of potential stress, pause, take a breath and try not to react automatically. Take a moment to think.
- Ask yourself: What am I reacting to? What do I think is going to happen here? Am I underestimating my ability to cope? Is there another way of looking at this? Is there another way of dealing with this?
- In general, try to face situations rather than avoid them. This can be done using a 'stepped approach': begin by putting yourself into your least feared situation until your anxiety reduces and then work upwards at a manageable pace until you reach the situation you fear the most.

If anxiety is persistent or interferes with everyday life, seek advice from your GP.

Third wave CBT

Over the last two decades, a 'third wave' of CBT has developed. Behaviour therapy in the early 20th century formed the first wave and Beck's cognitive therapy the second. Third wave CBT offers 'mindfulness' (Kabat-Zinn 2003) and 'acceptance' (Hayes *et al*. 2004) approaches, which include meditation practice and are influenced by Buddhist thinking. Rather than necessarily aiming to change the content of thoughts, people are encouraged to observe *how* they are thinking; in other words, it is suggested that they become more aware or more mindful of the way they think. People are encouraged to accept thoughts simply as mental processes and to be more tolerant and less judgemental about themselves in general. Mindfulness shares the CBT premise that thoughts are 'mental events' rather than facts (Teasdale *et al*. 2000) and that people should practise focusing on the 'here and now' rather than following anxious thinking patterns about the past or future. They might, for example, focus attention on breathing and the physical sensations that accompany this or on the task they are currently engaged with, paying attention to sensory aspects of the task that they might usually ignore. There is a growing body of evidence that mindfulness can be a helpful strategy for coping with both physical and mental health issues (Hofmann *et al*. 2010).

Acceptance and Commitment therapy takes this a step further and can be particularly beneficial for physical health issues; encouraging mindfulness and helping people to work towards meaningful goals alongside living with long-term health conditions have been found to be as effective as CBT with a range of mental and physical health issues (A-tjak *et al*. 2015).

We draw on aspects of mindfulness in the self-help guide: our breathing exercise shares similarities with 'mindful' breathing, and we encourage attention to breathing to be a cue for remaining in the present as a way of dealing with stress and hot flushes. The stress section and final session will also help you to re-engage with activities that are meaningful to you and using them as part of your coping strategy to manage menopausal transition.

Will CBT work for menopausal symptoms?

In the previous chapter we outlined the research on factors that influence hot flushes and night sweats. These included physiological mechanisms as well as psychological factors such as stress, thoughts and behaviours. Stress, for example, is an important factor that might increase the likelihood of experiencing a hot flush due to its impact on physiological systems, as well as through the effect it has on our ability to cope with hot flushes and night sweats. A CBT approach explains how the cognitive and emotional responses often reported during hot flushes can exacerbate the physical symptoms of a hot flush.

To illustrate how thinking can impact on how women feel emotionally and physically during a hot flush, what they do to try to cope and how these responses can then strengthen belief in the initial thought, let's look at an example of two different cognitive responses to a hot flush (Table 3.1).

Compare how the thinking (cognitive) responses of the two women can lead to very different consequences. Sue appraises the flush as threatening and completely out of her control. Consequently, she has a range of negative feelings, which arouse physiological responses, and she experiences the situation as very distressing. She is likely to start to feel anxious in public situations at the possibility of having a hot flush again, which,

Table 3.1 Two women's different reactions to hot flushes

	Sue	*Ann*
Situation	Hot flush starts in public place with heat building around chest, sudden increase in body temperature	
Thoughts	Oh no, not again; this is the last thing I need. I can't cope with this. People will notice. (negative beliefs about menopause and being in control)	This will pass in a minute – every woman goes through it. (neutral beliefs about menopause)
Emotions	Panic, anger/frustration, helpless, embarrassed, self-conscious.	Calm, acceptance.
Behaviour	Try and hide face, fan self frantically, leave room as quickly as possible.	Breathe through the flush until it passes, focus back on task, use humour if in company.
Physical	Flustered, palpitations, sweating, blushing, tense.	None other than hot flush symptoms.

over time, can begin to diminish her confidence and may lead her to begin to avoid things. Ann, on the other hand, does not experience her hot flush as a threatening event but a normal process that is part of the menopause transition and which will pass quickly. Her calm thinking style means that she remains calm in the situation which reinforces her initial calm response, leading her to maintain confidence and participation in daily life.

So what differentiates these two women? Is it that Ann's hot flushes are just less frequent than Sue's, and therefore she finds it easier to carry on with what she is doing without feeling distressed? Not necessarily. Research suggests that the factors that make hot flushes distressing are not entirely related to the frequency of the hot flushes; factors such as high daily stress levels and negative appraisals are also important (Rendall *et al.* 2008; Hanisch *et al.* 2008), as Ann and Sue's experiences illustrate. Therefore, as well as probably having varied life-styles and circumstances, Ann and Sue's differing approaches illustrate how hot flushes can be managed in a variety of ways.

The self-help guide in Chapters 4–7 will help you to under-stand your own experiences currently and generate ideas about how you can best manage hot flushes, night sweats and other symptoms. While the example in Table 3.1 makes these differences look clear cut and therefore easy to change, it is important not to underestimate how entrenched beliefs may be, and therefore the process of change may take time. While the self-help guide does not work at the level of core beliefs about ourselves, it can be helpful to think about how you view the menopause and ageing on the whole as they often go hand in hand. Consider how popular media such as news-papers, social media or television programmes tend to portray menopausal women and how this may influence your own feelings about menopause. These factors can have a direct or more indirect, subtle influence on your beliefs about yourself or about the menopause and may influence your responses to menopause-related symptoms.

Sue, for example, may have more negative beliefs about the menopause overall; she may remember her mother having a terrible time, or she may be more susceptible to negative media portrayals of menopausal women or have negative beliefs and assumptions about ageing – all too understandable in our youth-obsessed society. It can take time to process and change these influences, particularly if they have developed over a long period of time. Hot flushes can also undermine high standards for some women, which can mean that they harbour negative feelings about themselves. Sue may be so busy with various family or work commitments that she puts the needs of others before her own and subsequently gets no time to herself – which can lead to more stress. All of this takes time to change, and it is important that Sue makes small, manageable changes over a period, which is why the self-help guide is designed in weekly modules to work through, as you would do in formal therapy sessions.

Ann, by contrast, although exposed to negative media and cultural portrayals of menopausal or 'older' women, may dismiss them as overly negative and unhelpful and instead is more likely to focus on positive images of the mid-aged or 'older woman'. While she values her appearance, she may also be likely to recognise and hold other qualities in high esteem, such as achievements, positive personal characteristics and her relationships with family and friends. Ann may be generally less stressed because she makes sure that even though she has responsibilities for other family members, she makes sure that she makes time for herself to relax and views this time as being as important (if not more so!) than her other responsibilities.

If you think you are more likely to share Sue's response to hot flushes, the self-help guide will help you to identify factors that may be making a significant contribution to your current well-being and how you are coping generally. If you share Ann's response, that's great; the self-help guide will help you to understand why and how these views and reactions are helpful and hopefully offer some other ideas for you to add to your existing repertoire of positive coping behaviour.

Drawing on support from others

During this time, whether it is as you complete the self-help guide or more generally during the menopause transition, it can be helpful to consider additional sources of support rather than try to manage completely on your own. This can be by talking with friends going through menopause, talking to a partner and/or considering resources at work.

An interesting study by Liao et al. (2014) involved interviews with male partners of women going through menopause. Several themes arose highlighting partners as an important but under-utilised source of support. The men interviewed talked about observing their partners going through menopause and that they themselves viewed menopause as a period of transition. Importantly, they felt that this transition should be a shared process that required them to work together as a couple, but often they felt 'helpless' and 'redundant'. The barrier reported was that they considered the subject of menopause to be comparable to periods in terms of the 'etiquette' involved; i.e. that it is generally rarely discussed and certainly not in detail. Men were concerned that if they raised the subject with their partners, this may cause distress, and this was compounded by a general lack of information available about menopause and their own awareness of their lack of knowledge. This study highlights how the 'taboo' nature of the subject of menopause prevents couples from communicating with their partners and in turn accessing potential valuable support.

With this in mind, there are a couple of useful books that have been written specifically for men on the subject of meno-pause. The first is Ruth Devlin's *Men . . . Let's Talk Menopause*, which takes an evidence-based and often humorous approach, aimed at understanding menopause symptoms, why they occur and what can help; a more general evidence-based book for women and men is Kathy Abernethy's *Menopause: The One-Stop Guide* (see References).

Some larger work places have begun to have workshops to raise awareness about menopause, and some women are starting to set up their own support groups at work. There is guidance available for organisations about how to provide a 'menopause-friendly workplace' and what practical support might be available (Trades Union Congress (TUC), Faculty of Occupational Medicine (FOM) and Chartered Institute of Personnel and Development (CIPD)) (see Resources).

Social media has provided support and contacts for many women; for example, 'Menopause Cafés' have sprung up around the UK providing support and the opportunity to talk about menopause (see Resources). Moreover, involving a partner or friend in your self-help CBT for hot flushes could provide you with additional support and encouragement – you could also join up with friends to work through the following chapters together or form a WhatsApp group as some women we worked with have enjoyed doing.

Managing menopausal hot flushes and night sweats

A four-week self-help guide

Hot flush rating scale

Before you start: You can rate your hot flushes so that you can see whether they change at the end of the four weeks.

1 **How often have you had hot flushes in the past week?**
Please estimate: 20. times each day or . . . times each week

2 **If you have night sweats, how often have they woken you up in the past week?**
Please estimate: 3. . times each day, or . . . times each week

Please circle a number on each scale to indicate how your flushes/sweats have been during the past week:

3 **To what extent do you regard your flushes/sweats as a problem?**
No problem at all   Very much a problem

1 2 3 4 5 6 7 8 9 (10)

4 **How distressed do you feel about your hot flushes?**
Not distressed at all   Very distressed indeed

1 2 3 4 5 6 (7) 8 9 10

5 **How much do your hot flushes interfere with your daily routine?**
Not at all   Very much indeed

1 2 3 4 5 6 (7) 8 9 10

Add up the numbers of hot flushes and night sweats in the past week which gives your

Hot flush frequency total score = . 23 . .

and add up the scores on numbers 3, 4 and 5 and divide by 3. This will give you your

Problem-rating score = . . . 8 . . .

Introduction and outline of the self-help guide

This four-week self-help guide is designed to help you to understand and manage your menopausal symptoms, taking in to account the range of factors that have been shown to influence women's experience of menopause in Chapters 1 and 2. We will be summarizing some of the information from these chapters briefly so that the self-help guide can be read as a stand-alone section. We have found that this treatment approach can help women going through the natural menopause transition as well as those who have menopausal symptoms triggered by surgery or medical treatments, such as treatments for breast cancer.

Menopause is a time of transition during which we are often confronted by changes in our bodies and sometimes in the way we think about ourselves. There is no doubt that in our society, this time of midlife can be challenging as we strive to balance the needs of others – such as children still at home or leaving home or elderly parents needing more care – as well as work and other responsibilities. You may also have a feeling of 'now or never' about plans you have been hoping to pursue but never seem to have gotten around to because of other demands. This guide is designed to help you to manage the key physical symptoms of the menopause, hot flushes and night sweats, as well as providing information on promoting well-being and general good health during this time in your life. For some women the menopause can be a welcome occurrence, as it means the end of menstruation, the need for contraception and the possibility of pregnancy. At the same time, there can be feelings of loss or concerns about health and uncertainty about what lies ahead. Worries about ageing can be a factor too, especially in a society that places a high value on youth and youthful beauty. You may encounter negative attitudes towards the menopause and menopausal women, or even find you hold some yourself.

What thoughts come to mind when you think of 'menopause'? If you write them down here, we can look back at them at the end of the programme:

. . . .
. . . .
. . . .

If you find that your thoughts around menopause are based on negative assumptions around inevitable decline, hopefully this book will help you to begin to question their validity. It can be helpful to view menopause as a time to reassess your life and consider the opportunities for your own development and lifestyle. Using this guide and undertaking the relaxation, goal-setting and other activities can help you to accept and approach the changes that are taking place. As a result, you can gain some control over your menopause experience and improve your well-being.

What is involved?

This guide provides information and strategies that you can use to deal with menopausal symptoms. It is based on CBT, which is widely used by psychologists and others to help people deal with a variety of emotional and physical health problems, such as anxiety, stress, pain and sleep-related issues. A summary of how CBT can help these problems can be found in Chapter 3. CBT helps people to explore the way that they think (cognitive) and behave and make changes as necessary in order to feel better and cope more effectively with symptoms. CBT is used throughout the programme and particularly in the sections on stress, dealing with hot flushes, night sweats and sleep.

The main components of the self-help guide include:

- being informed about menopausal symptoms;
- understanding what can help you cope with your symptoms;
- learning to use relaxation and paced breathing;
- taking steps to reduce general levels of stress;
- identifying and modifying triggers of hot flushes;
- dealing with negative thoughts and behavioural reactions;
- practising relaxation and breathing at the onset of a flush;
- dealing with hot flushes in social situations; and
- managing night sweats and sleep.

The guide also includes a web link to breathing and relaxation audio instructions.

We will be providing an example of how one woman used the self-help guide. Our case study is Jane, and you will be able to see how she applied the workbook to her own situation in the chapters that follow.

How to use this guide

- This is a four-week self-help guide that should help you to deal with and reduce the negative impact of hot flushes and night sweats.

- Our research has found that this treatment helps women to manage menopausal symptoms, and we hope that you will find it useful as well.
- The self-help aspect of this guide means that you will learn skills to help you manage the symptoms yourself. With practice and commitment, these skills will improve over time and can be integrated into everyday life. Women we have worked with report that it is the practice outside of sessions that really made the difference (rather than just reading through the guide).
- Choose a four-week period during which you set aside a one-hour 'treatment session' each week.
- The programme is set out in four discrete sections so that you can read through and then plan your own weekly programme.
- Your weekly programme will usually include relaxation with the audio instructions, as well as practising the management of hot flushes and night sweats. You can download the audio instructions for relaxation and paced breathing from the eResources site: www.routledge.com/9780367853037 Women found it helpful to copy the instructions onto a CD, smartphone or MP3 player so that they can listen to them whenever they choose, day or night.
- Each week will build on what you have learned and practised in the previous week, so it is important to complete the whole self-help guide in order, even if you feel the main issue for you is dealt with in a later chapter.
- You will be asked to complete a daily diary, which you'll find at the end of each chapter in the guide, so that you can monitor your flushes as well as your homework. So after reading the guide for each week, you can fill in the diary and put the homework into practice.

Good luck!

4

Week 1

Being informed and reducing stress

Getting started: being informed and making time for yourself

This is Week 1 of the self-help guide. We'll begin by focusing on information about menopause as well as on some relaxation and breathing exercises. Getting the most out of the programme will be down to you. Sometimes it can be difficult to set aside time for ourselves, so before we go any further, think about how you might be able to fit the programme into everyday life. To put the information and advice into practice and to learn new skills, you will need to set aside about 30 minutes each day and another hour each week for the next four weeks. A diary is included at the end of each week, and you can use this to monitor changes in your hot flushes as well as to record homework tasks.

Many women put the needs of others first, so it may be challenging to find time for yourself in the beginning. You may even feel as though you are stealing time from something or someone else, but we would strongly recommend you allow yourself this time and space. Undertaking the relaxation exercises and other tasks in the guide will make you feel more accepting and in control of what is happening to you and is likely to have some positive effects on other parts of your life as well. Be patient too – try not to get discouraged if you find it hard initially or don't experience change immediately. It will take time and practice to discover what works best for you within a self-management approach. If you miss one or two days, it doesn't mean you have to start again – don't give up. Simply decide that today will be different and be determined to find the time.

Committing yourself to working on your own needs is worthwhile and ultimately rewarding. Our work with women in the past has shown that even small changes can make a big difference. In this guide we have included many comments from women who have taken part in this treatment because they provide an additional and helpful perspective.

What is the menopause?

On average the first signs of menopause, such as changes in menstruation or hot flushes, occur in our mid- to-late 40s, but there is wide variation between women. A woman is considered postmenopausal when she has not menstruated for 12 months. For some women, however, the menopause happens suddenly as the result of surgery or of taking certain medications. For women who have had breast cancer, menopausal symptoms may be yet another thing to deal with at a time when they have already undergone a difficult treatment regime and are trying to get their lives back on track or come to terms with how their illness has affected them.

The menopause is not necessarily a problematic time, but it occurs during midlife when you may be dealing with other life challenges, such as parents' ill health or bereavement, adolescent children, children leaving home (or not leaving home!), work demands or simply reassessing life in middle age. As with other times of physical and psychological transition, such as adolescence or having a first child, these are all normal processes, but they can feel overwhelming at times. It can help to deal with each area separately, and, most of all, it is important to have time to think and to process these changes. Most changes can have both positive and negative aspects, but it helps to notice the potential benefits.

Recent studies have shown that the menopause can be difficult for about 25 per cent of women (mainly because of troublesome hot flushes and night sweats). However, studies of women across the age range suggest that after the menopause, women often have more energy and increased feelings of well-being.

What are menopausal symptoms?

The physical symptoms most commonly experienced during the menopause are hot flushes and night sweats, which affect on average 60 to 70 per cent of women during the natural menopause. Approximately 25 per cent of women report having troublesome hot flushes that interfere with their quality of life. And, as described in Chapter 2, these symptoms can be more severe following a sudden menopause, such as that following surgery or breast cancer treatments, for example. They are usually described as sudden sensations of heat that spread to the upper body, but they do vary considerably between women. Shivering also happens. The flushes can be accompanied by sweating and palpitations, understandably causing discomfort and disrupting sleep. Hot flushes and night sweats are the main specific physical symptoms experienced during the menopause. By becoming informed about these, you can pass on this information to your friends and family – these symptoms need not be thought of as shameful or embarrassing.

Some women feel low in mood and anxious during the menopause, and the tiredness and disturbed sleep that accompany night sweats and flushes can certainly contribute to this. Women are also having to cope with the stresses and strains of everyday life as they try to combat these symptoms. However, depression is not necessarily part of the menopause, and many of the other symptoms attributed to this transitional life stage are caused by other events in our lives or general ageing. Negative views about the menopause and menopausal women can also unconsciously affect our self-esteem. It can be useful to challenge unhelpful assumptions about the menopause and about ageing, and we hope that this book will help you to do this.

For women who have had breast cancer, low mood and anxiety can be part of coming to terms with the experience of being diagnosed with, and having treatment for, this illness. However, if these feelings begin to interfere significantly with your everyday life, visit your GP and ask for a referral to more specialist psychological support services.

Hot flushes are sometimes associated with concentration and memory-related problems. Again, disrupted sleep can affect your memory, as can having too much to do. Research studies do not show a particular association between a natural menopause and memory – we all forget more with age. But if we are feeling anxious, low or stressed, our attention (and therefore our memory) are affected. This happens to people of all ages. The best strategy is to try not to worry about it and to focus on the things that you need to remember by writing them down.

What causes menopausal symptoms?

Hot flushes occur when our body is adjusting to declining levels of oestrogen during the menopause transition. Flushes tend to be more frequent when oestrogen reduces rapidly; this can happen following surgical menopause and is also common following courses of chemotherapy or hormone treatment (such as tamoxifen) for breast cancer. Once the body gradually adjusts to having lower levels of oestrogen, menopausal symptoms tend to tail off. Some women might be more prone to hot flushes than others: in large-scale studies, women who smoke tend to report more hot flushes, while those who exercise more regularly tend to have fewer. However, it is still difficult to predict which woman will have troublesome hot flushes on an individual basis.

Hormone levels affect our body temperature control mechanisms during the menopause; it is as though our internal 'thermostat' has a narrower range, and so our bodies try to cool down by having a hot flush in response to small temperature increases, in our bodies or in our surroundings. As well as changes in oestrogen, higher levels of general stress can also increase the likelihood of hot flushes occurring (see Figure 4.1).

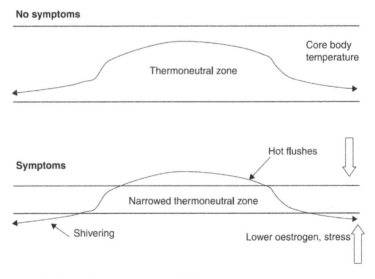

Figure 4.1 The thermoneutral zone (TNZ) and hot flushes: showing core body temperature fluctuations within the TNZ for women without hot flushes (no symptoms) and the narrowed TNZ for women with hot flush symptoms

Source: Adapted and reproduced with kind permission from Archer *et al.* (2011)

What happens during a hot flush?

Figure 4.1 shows what actually happens during a hot flush. Core body temperature varies within a 'thermoneutral zone', or hot flush 'threshold', which is narrowed when oestrogen levels reduce. It can also be lowered by stress. The top part of the diagram shows a woman without hot flushes. Her core body temperature can vary within the zone without causing any symptoms. The woman represented in the lower part of the diagram has a narrowed thermoneutral zone, and for her, small changes in body temperature cause flushing or shivering. Flushes can be triggered by internal or external events such as temperature changes, anxiety or even hot food and caffeine.

> I think that I've been having quite a few hot flushes lately because my mother has been ill, a friend collapsed at work . . . you know, there were lots of enormous things. So just the fact that I can think 'well, there is a reason for me getting more hot and bothered' is helpful.

> I'd have these flushes . . . when I'd been rushing, like in the morning. I'm thinking now let's prioritize, get myself ready, get myself up a little bit earlier and prepare myself so I don't get into a rush.

This is why relaxation is important. Relaxation and paced breathing can reduce general stress levels and may reduce the impact of flushes when they occur.

There is some evidence that the way we think about, and react to, flushes can make a difference. Dealing with thoughts and behaviours will also be part of this self-help programme.

Understanding hot flushes: a cognitive behavioural approach

Figure 4.2 shows how hot flushes and night sweats are influenced by bodily changes (such as fluctuating hormone levels and hot flush threshold) but also by stress and lifestyle factors as well as thoughts, emotions and behaviours. For example, one woman might think that people are looking at her critically when she has hot flushes, causing her to cut back on socializing with others (behavioural reaction); she might then feel worse about herself, however, and become more stressed (emotional reaction).

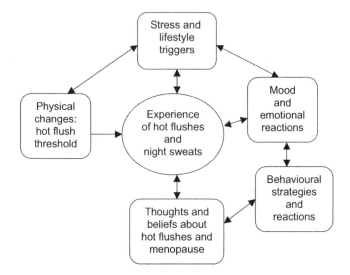

Figure 4.2 A cognitive behavioural model of hot flushes

Source: Adapted and reproduced with permission from Hunter (2003)

> [I was] really embarrassed and thinking that people were watching me, and yet I was drawing attention to myself. The emotions were making things much, much worse. And the more stressed I got when a flush started, the worse the flush would actually be.

Compare this to another woman who doesn't think that others notice or doesn't really care if they do. She would continue to meet people as part of her daily life (positive behaviour), and having a hot flush would not make her feel stressed or uncomfortable around other people.

> I never did find them a big problem socially or anything. I just get on with it because all the women around me are doing the same thing anyway.

> I get hot at times but it doesn't bother me. If it's hot, I just open the window but otherwise I don't have any ill effects at all.

These examples show how our reactions in terms of our thoughts, what we do (behaviour) and how we feel (emotions) can affect our experience of hot flushes. As we have learned, unhelpful reactions can increase the likelihood that hot flushes will have a negative impact on our lives.

Relaxation and breathing

Relaxation involves learning a skill – you get better at it the more you do it, so it helps to practise every day by listening to the audio recording at a regular time and place for 10 to 15 minutes.

Find a comfortable chair in a quiet room and tell other people that you need a quarter of an hour to yourself, without interruptions. Don't try too hard; just listen and follow the instructions as best you can. Your mind may wander from time to time, but just bring your attention slowly back to the relaxation practice and what is happening in your body and in your thoughts. Over time, your relaxation skills will develop.

The recording includes a relaxation and paced breathing practice. We recommend you start off by listening to the relaxation and breathing practice every day, so that you learn how to relax your body and follow your breathing. Focusing on slow-paced breathing from your stomach (known as 'diaphragmatic' breathing; see Box 4.1) is helpful for a number of reasons:

1 Breathing slows down your body's responses, especially when you are stressed, which will help you reach a calmer state.
2 If practised regularly, diaphragmatic breathing can help to improve overall well-being.
3 You can do the practice any time.
4 It can be a useful cue for general relaxation if you are feeling stressed.
5 If you are experiencing a hot flush, breathing focuses your attention away from the flush and onto something else.

Box 4.1 Paced breathing

Paced breathing is slow, even breathing from your stomach. It is also known as 'diaphragmatic' breathing. The diaphragm is located just below the lungs and forms a barrier between them and the stomach. Breathing from the stomach, or below the diaphragm, means that we get more oxygen because pushing the diaphragm down increases lung capacity. Practising diaphragmatic breathing means keeping the chest and shoulders still and pushing the stomach out, all the while taking slower, deeper breaths. Putting one hand on your chest and one hand on your stomach helps as you get used to this way of breathing. Try to keep the hand on your chest still, and the hand on your stomach should rise and fall in line with your breaths. It might be easier to practise this lying down at first, but once you get the hang of it, you'll be able to use this breathing in many parts of your daily life.

It is portable – it's not something that you've got to do at a certain time in a certain place. It's not like taking a pill where you're going to need a glass of water; you can just start deep breathing and switching off wherever.

Women who took part in our studies of hot flushes tended to view paced breathing as one of the most helpful strategies because it could potentially be applied in any situation. They also felt that they were more able to cope with the flushes they did experience. Remember, this can take practice and may not work immediately, but we found that women we worked with reported more improvement the more they practised.

I thought the relaxation actually worked and it worked because I did it every single day for that 10–15 minutes.

When you feel a flush coming on, you can apply the relaxation response by relaxing your shoulders and arms, focusing on your breathing and letting the flush flow over you.

Sometimes I will just stop for a while and actually focus on my breathing. That's one of my first ports of call . . . to just take a deep breath and to tell myself to calm down. So I do that quite a lot and I can do that anywhere. I can sit down on the train and close my eyes and breathe in and out and nobody would know that I'm doing relaxation. . . . I'm able to just shut my mind off from what's going on around me.

Don't fight the hot flush – accept it and breathe through it.

Homework

- Practise relaxation exercises every day if possible (or for at least five out of every seven days) and mark this by putting an X in your weekly diary when you practise.

Reducing hot flush triggers

Studies of women with menopausal symptoms suggest that about 50 per cent of flushes may be triggered by particular events. These might include eating spicy foods, drinking hot drinks or alcohol, rushing or a rapid change in temperature. We have found that these triggers vary widely between women; in fact, some women can't identify any triggers at all. It is worth looking for any particular behaviours or lifestyle factors that trigger hot flushes for you, though.

> When I was in the car and somebody pulled out in front of me . . . adrenaline would trigger it. That could be quite quick. Also, very quick changes in temperature would also trigger it. . .

> The minute I have a hot cup of tea that can bring it on, so I've reduced the amount of tea that I drink . . . well, any hot drink, to be honest. I don't drink hot drinks at night any more. I know what the triggers are now so I avoid them.

Keeping a diary (see the homework section at the end of Week 1) can enable you to identify triggers. By making small lifestyle changes, you might then be able to gain some control over your menopausal symptoms.

> I started to realize that there were changes I could make, [such as] having a fan, opening windows, wearing layers. You need to think, 'OK, this is what's going on and this is what I need to do to change it'.

So this week, as well as recording hot flushes and night sweats in the weekly diary, try to identify what brings on a flush or sweat for you by thinking about what was happening just before the flush began. You might also notice general patterns in your diary. For example, some women notice that their flushes are worse in the evenings or when they are tired; they may also notice that the flushes are *less* frequent when they are engaged in particular activities. The diary can be very helpful in understanding your hot flush patterns, and this is the first step towards managing them.

> I now know that everything that can make you feel better is worth bothering about. It was just like 'Urgh, it's going to be like this and I'm just going to have to put up with it' and actually no, take some steps and actually do something about it.

Try not to feel discouraged if you can't find any specific triggers. Remember only half of flushes tend to have a clear trigger and this tends to vary between individuals. Chapter 4 will help you to think about strategies to manage the flushes when they occur even if you can't identify triggers.

Box 4.2

Jane is a 53-year-old woman who was diagnosed with breast cancer three years ago. She has been treated successfully with a combination of surgery, chemotherapy and radiotherapy and now takes tamoxifen. Jane has hot flushes and night sweats that range in intensity from mild to severe, and she generally carries a fan around with her, although often feels embarrassed about using it in company. She also wears layers that can easily be removed during and after a flush to help her cool down. Jane noticed that her triggers included drinking coffee (five cups per day) and stress. As a first step, she decided to reduce her coffee intake and drink tea or water instead of coffee in the afternoons.

Homework

- Keep a daily diary recording hot flushes and night sweats and make a note of any triggers.

Stress and lifestyle factors

As we enter our midlife period, life can be very busy, and a raft of changes can occur. Many women find they are juggling teenage children, elderly parents, work and relationships with families and friends. And you may be trying to make time for new activities and interests. In addition, the changes you are experiencing in your own body may be causing you stress or occupying your thoughts. With so much going on, it can be difficult to remember that we need to keep our own needs in mind.

Well, I feel OK about myself; it's other people's attitudes that I find difficult.

It suddenly makes you think, 'God I'm 50, where has my life gone?'

For women who have experienced breast cancer diagnosis and treatment, ongoing worries or simply coming to terms with the emotional and physical impact of treatment can be an additional burden. It is particularly important that during times of stress you take care of yourself. The rest of this chapter will consider ways you can take better care of yourself to manage these feelings and improve your well-being overall.

It can be useful to remember that taking care of yourself doesn't mean becoming selfish. It will, however, enable you to participate more fully in all aspects of life. For a start, you'll have more energy and be more relaxed when problems or stressful situations arise, and you'll be able to deal with these more effectively. The following section will give information about stress, what happens when it affects us, and a range of strategies for managing it. While you may not find all of the strategies helpful, and you may not feel stressed at all, this section is designed to help you to tailor an individual plan to reduce stress or equally to increase well-being.

There are so many strands – ageing, sexuality, thinking about the past and future, then there's your mother, your work, everyone reacting to you. It's not just one thing.

Dealing with stress

It's important to remember that stress is a normal and unavoidable part of everyday life. However, what is considered stressful varies from person to person. Something may bother you, yet another woman may seem to take it in her stride. At the same time, you can probably identify situations and experiences that you cope with well but which others might find stressful.

I don't worry about things I can't change. I've always been a little bit like that. What is the point in stressing about something that I can't change? The things I can change, I do try to work on, I really don't get terribly stressed about things.

Stress usually happens when we are in a situation that seems too demanding or overwhelming, and we think that we don't have the personal resources to deal with it: we start to think that we can't cope. And that's the nub of the issue: how we think about events and ourselves makes a difference to how stressful we find them.

The body's response to any threat is called the 'fight or flight response'. This is a primitive survival mechanism during which the body is primed to respond to danger by either fighting it or running away (flight). When we feel under threat, the body releases adrenaline to quickly send blood and oxygen to the muscles so that they are prepared for action. Our breathing becomes faster in order to take in more oxygen, and muscles tense to help the body fight or run. This response was very useful for our survival thousands of years ago but is not as useful in modern life as our bodies are unable to distinguish between life-threatening dangers and everyday worries such as being late or pressure at work. If you have many demands in your daily life, this stress response can be constantly activated. While this is not dangerous – and in some situations stress can actually be helpful as it makes us more alert and generally 'on the ball' – over time, it can lead to a range of physical and psychological consequences. Signs of stress fall under four main categories:

1 physical signs (fight or flight response), such as butterflies in your stomach or a racing heart;
2 emotional signs, such as feeling worried, low or angry;
3 behavioural signs, such as withdrawing from people or sleeping more or less than usual; and
4 cognitive (thinking) signs, such as thoughts along the lines of 'I'll never get this done!', 'I'm not good enough!' or 'I can't please everyone!'

These emotional, behavioural and cognitive signs tend to occur when we experience stress over an extended period or when we experience small everyday stresses frequently and don't take time to relax.

The vicious cycle

These different reactions to stress all influence each other. For example, if you think negatively, you are more likely to have negative emotions, experience physical symptoms of stress and behave in a 'stressed' way. This is called a 'vicious cycle' (see Figure 4.3) as once you are feeling more stressed, emotionally and physically, you are then more likely to believe any overly negative thoughts.

Finding ways to tackle negative thinking and behaviour can help you feel calmer, even in stressful situations. Given

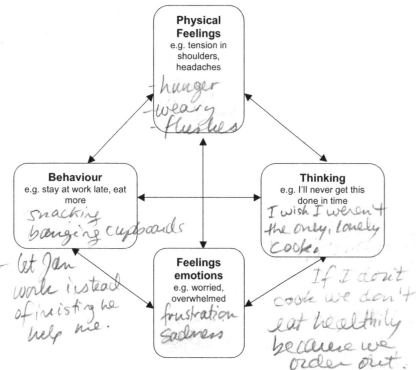

Figure 4.3 The vicious cycle: cognitive behavioural reactions to stress

A printable copy of this figure is available to download; visit the 'eResources' site: www.routledge.com/9780367853037

the impact that stress can have on hot flushes, reducing stress is one of the first steps you can take to help you to cope with flushes and reduce their impact on your daily life. To begin with, it's important to recognise the signs that indicate you are becoming stressed.

What might be stressful for you? It may be helpful to think of the last time you felt stressed. Note down a situation that you find stressful (e.g. at work or at home):

Getting dinner on the table when tired + hungry.

Look at Figure 4.3 again and think about your reactions to one of the stressful situations that you have noted here. Can you identify your 'stress signs'? Write down your stress signs, i.e. physical feelings, thinking, feelings/emotions and behaviour, in Figure 4.3.

> With my boss at work I do feel stressed when I have too much to do. I worry and often work late. It's at those times I can feel overwhelmed and that's when I feel the hot flushes come.

In the example shown in Figure 4.3, the stressful situation that makes this woman worried and overwhelmed is her heavy workload. The reason she feels worried and overwhelmed is due to the negative way she is thinking about the situation: 'I won't finish the task in time' and 'My colleagues might disapprove'. She is making predictions about what will happen in the future and *expecting* everything to go wrong. Although this is potentially a valid perspective on the situation, this woman is not considering any alternative views of it because she is stressed. This thinking style will not only lead to negative emotions but will also have an impact on her behaviour – she is staying late at work and experiencing physical consequences in the form of tension and headaches. Working longer hours is making her even more stressed and irritable and reinforcing her worries about getting the task finished. The vicious cycle is in place.

Managing stressful situations

Finding ways to tackle negative thinking and behaviour can help you to feel calmer even in stressful situations or when you are having a hot flush. This is particularly important, as we know that stress can make flushes worse. Slowing down your breathing and stopping to think for a few moments before you react can be a helpful first step to managing stress. These strategies can also give you space to choose how best to respond to stressful thinking or even pick up that you are falling into that rut:

> At work I get so busy that I snap when someone asks me to do yet another trivial thing. . . . [U]sing the breathing helped me to stop and think about that person who has just spoken to me . . . and to stop for a moment and respond more calmly.

The first step to changing stressed thinking is to notice that it is there in the first place – we all do it at times! Don't worry if you had difficulty writing down any thoughts in the space on page 93, as they can be tricky to identify. One way to spot stressed or anxious thinking is to consider what you are expecting to happen in a given situation, as it is often this that is making you feel stressed. It may be that you are overestimating the chance that things will go wrong – this is anxious thinking. We do not necessarily notice specific thoughts, but instead we can be aware of a critical inner voice that is hurrying us to rush around or predicting disaster: for example, 'What did I do that for? I look really stupid now!'

It will be helpful if you can become more aware of the way you are thinking over the next week. When you are feeling a bit stressed, pay attention to your inner voice and see if any common themes arise. The more you are able to practise identifying thoughts or thought patterns, the easier it becomes; the next section includes ideas that can help you to work towards a calmer approach to everyday life.

> Changing your thinking is something that you're not conscious of and it's something that you have to watch. And that doesn't change overnight. . . . [T]here are days when you are going to feel sad. What I say to myself is 'these are only thoughts . . . I don't have to react to them'. And once I start talking myself through it, I think, 'who's leading me, am I leading my mind or is my mind leading me?'

Stressful thoughts are just one view of a situation. They tend to represent a very anxious or negative view, however, and they can have a real impact on how we feel about that situation. If we think stressful, anxious or catastrophic thoughts, our stress and anxiety levels can rocket! Having a more helpful, calmer or accepting view of the situation can make you feel calmer and therefore more able to respond (behave) in a neutral way.

Unhelpful thoughts	Helpful thoughts
'I'll never get this done'.	'Even if I don't get everything done, it's not the end of the world'.
'I'm no good'.	'Everyone has ups and downs; it doesn't mean I'm no good'.

This can take practice as often when we *are* stressed, we find it extremely difficult to consider calmer approaches!

Living in London and commuting . . . all that is stressful. But what I've tried to do is 'change the channel' in my head. I changed my thoughts. If I'm getting stressed, I try to watch for when I can feel my stress levels coming up. . . . And then, you know, just watch myself, and say 'now calm down', and just talk myself through it.

Box 4.3

Jane works in a senior role as a nurse in a busy hospital and constantly felt behind with her workload as junior nurses approached her with queries and questions frequently during the day. She often felt unable to delegate tasks and would often take time away from her own job to help them out. She completed the cognitive behavioural model of her stress:

- Thoughts: If I don't do it, they will do it wrong.
- Feelings: Stress, frustration, anxiety.
- Behaviour: Does other people's tasks. Allows herself to be constantly interrupted.
- Physiological: Hot flushes, palpitations, tension, poor sleep.

Jane identified that her beliefs about other people's abilities had a direct effect on her stress and her behaviour. By constantly acting as though this thought were true, she never gave herself or others a chance to test it and perhaps prove otherwise.

Dealing with stressful thinking

Looking again now at Figure 4.3 and what you have written in the thinking box ('Thinking'), run through the following questions to help you find a calmer approach to your stressful situation. Don't worry about finding answers to all of the questions; even filling in just a few may help you to look at the situation differently and therefore feel less stressed.

1 Is my way of thinking helping me to cope with the situation?
Yes/No

If yes, how is it helpful?

....
....

If no, how is it unhelpful?

Jan can't read my mind. Take out food can be healthy sometimes.

2 Would a friend agree completely with my perspective of the situation? (In our example, would a friend agree and say, 'You'll never get that done; everyone will think badly of you!' or might he or she have a different perspective? A calm friend or colleague may point out that you generally *do* get things done in the end. He or she may also point out that you are well respected at work.)

Write down what a calm friend might say or do instead:

Ask Jan to make time to help with meals.

....

3 Imagine a friend in the same situation, feeling just as stressed. Would you agree with her catastrophic thinking, or would you offer her more calming words of advice to help her to deal with the situation? What would you say to her? *She is not failing her family. Talk to spouse about sharing responsibilities of cooking.*

In our example, it is likely that you would offer reassurance to a friend rather than criticism.

4 Now, taking these answers into account, write down a calmer thought in response to your stressful situation:

Maybe, if I ask, Jan will help me in the kitchen more often. It could be fun and I wouldn't feel the burden (constant) of keeping us healthy.

This is not simply positive thinking, but rather a way of taking a step back from the situation and viewing it from a more neutral and rational perspective. We know this is difficult to do when emotions are running high, but it is likely that your emotions/feelings will also change, and as a result, you may well feel less stressed. When we feel less tense or anxious, our behaviour is also calmer and less reactive, and we cope better. The main aim here is to develop a calmer, self-supportive approach rather than believing everything the 'voice of doom' in your head may say! Again, this skill must be learned, and you'll need to practise. The more you do so, the easier it will become to notice and question unhelpful thinking.

> You can often stand back from your friend's situation and say 'well, if you did so and so, then that would be helpful' or 'that would be a solution'. . . . I think taking a more analytical approach – 'what could we do about this?' or 'we've done as much as we can' – is helpful.

Finding calmer ways to behave

By transforming your stressful and unhelpful thinking to calmer, more constructive thoughts, it is likely that you will feel less stressed. You can also identify coping behaviours that will be more helpful.

Note down here what you tend to do when you feel stressed (e.g. eating too much, avoiding doing things or doing too much, withdrawing from certain people or activities, going to bed, drinking alcohol, etc.):

Withdrawing from people/activities
Going outside for walk or sit in garden

Next, make a list of what you do that makes you feel calm or content on a typical day, however small those things might be (e.g. going for a walk, exercise, calling a friend, having a cup of tea, reading a book):

Cooking, baking, sewing, watching
a good program.

Homework

Try to do more of the activities you find calming and pleasant, even for just a short time every day. Also find something specific that you can plan to do at a particular time – it really does make a difference to add a few positive activities to your routine. In addition, research shows that writing down three things that went well at the end of each day (however small) can lift mood and improve well-being. Why not try this and see if it works for you?

Problem-solving

If you have a particular practical problem to solve, give yourself a definite time in which to consider it and then follow the chart here to seek the best solution. Remember that you are looking for the best possible option, not a perfect solution.

First of all, identify the problem. Try to write a short summary of it, drawing out the main aspects of the situation and how it makes you feel (for example, 'When I am looking after my elderly parent on my own, I feel stressed out and angry because nobody else is helping out or taking responsibility').

Cooking dinner makes me feel frustrated + alone.

What would you like to change? Think about what would need to change in the situation for you to feel better about it. This may be your thinking or approach to it, or it may be a specific element of the situation that is stressful, such as others expecting too much of you.

Ian could help but tends to be working at that time of day.

What are your options? Brainstorm all possible solutions to the problem, however small or insignificant they may seem. Write them down here:

Ask for help at 5pm.
Ask for help earlier to prepare.

What has helped in the past? If you have been through similar situations before, did you find any course of action particularly useful?

....
....

Who might help?

... *Jan* ....

....

Pros and cons of each option:

... *It is hard for Jan to stop working* ....

... *He has flexible hours.* ....

....

Which seems the best option to try first?

... *Preparing food ahead of meal* ...

....

Make an action plan:

... *Talk it over.* ....

... *Use an alarm.* ....

Finally, review the situation: you might need to try another if the first option does not work as well as hoped.

For example, Sheila's problem was that she could not find any time for herself. She decided that to make more time, she would need her family, particularly her teenage children, to be more proactive around the house. She had tried nagging them (without success), so she planned to discuss this with her husband and with her sister, who had older children. She brainstormed options and decided the best one to start with was to have a family meeting. She and her husband helped the teenagers set goals that would enable them to become more independent and to take more responsibility for themselves – the first being to use their own alarm clocks to get up on time in the morning. Even a small change like this seemed to ease the pressure!

Pacing activities

When we are stressed, we often try to do too much and end up exhausting ourselves completely. We then need to rest but usually become even more stressed about what we are now not doing, so when our energy returns, we go full throttle and exhaust ourselves again. This is called the 'boom and bust' cycle. In Figure 4.4, the undulating black line represents fluctuating energy levels in the boom and bust cycle.

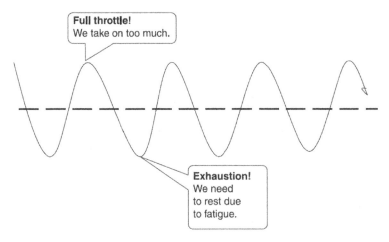

Figure 4.4 Boom and bust cycle

Falling into such a pattern of behaviour may be more likely to happen if you are recovering from a major period of stress or illness and are keen to 'get back to normal'. This may be particularly important to you if you have recently had treatment for breast cancer. The key to breaking the cycle is to stick to moderate levels of activity every day and to give yourself regular breaks (represented by the dashed line in Figure 4.4). This means resisting the temptation to do as much as possible, as you will be less likely to wear yourself out. People often find that when they adopt this approach, they actually get *more* done and feel less tired as well.

Another pacing strategy is to break down large, overwhelming tasks that you never get around to starting into a series of small steps and then doing each step one at a time with a break in between. This can be used at work (by breaking a project into small steps and ticking them off as you go, for example) or home (starting with clearing out one cupboard in a room rather than approaching the whole room as one job). By breaking big tasks down in this way, it is easier to make a start, and everything feels more manageable. Even if you have not completed the whole task in one day, you can do a few more steps tomorrow and will actually get the job done more quickly.

I do recognize that there are things outside your control, you know, and you need to focus on the things that you can change. I do that by making lists and breaking the list down because there's only so many things you're supposed to have on a list . . . and I reward myself for things you know [laughs].

Now, I just say, 'you can only do so much, delegate to the husband' [laughs]. If I can't get it done, I'll just shove it to one side and I'll get back to it another day. And I always have 'down time' which I never allowed myself before. . . . I find that a big comfort.

Box 4.4

Jane worked through the thinking questions and also used problem-solving to identify an alternative coping strategy that would help her reduce stress. Her answers to the thought questions were as follows:

1 *Is my way of thinking helping me to cope with the situation?* No.
If no, how is it unhelpful?
I am doing everyone else's jobs as well as my own!
2 *Would a friend agree completely with my perspective of the situation?*
No, they would probably advise me to tell people what to do and trust them to get on with it.
3 *Imagine a friend in the same situation feeling just as stressed. What would you say to her?*
I would advise her to delegate and to make time for herself to focus on her tasks.
4 *Now taking these answers into account, write down a calmer thought in response to your stressful situation:*

I can try to trust other people's capabilities to do their own jobs and take steps to protect my own time so I can concentrate on my own work.

This led to a (tentative) change of approach, which required Jane to 'test out' the alternative perspective and try out a different behaviour. She identified this using the problem-solving approach. The following week, she answered people's questions and then left them to get on with their work. Jane also put a sign

up on her office door for an hour each day request-
ing that she not be disturbed. She felt anxious about
this as she began thinking that the sign 'would be
ignored' but found to her surprise that giving others instructions enabled them to carry out their
tasks without any difficulty, and in turn they asked
fewer questions as they became more confident in
their own roles. She learned that staff respected her
request for peace and that she then felt less stressed
as she was on top of her workload. She also tried to
take the occasional break for ten minutes or so, even
if she was busy, and noticed she felt calmer and more
in control.

In summary

Helpful strategies

- Prioritizing your health and well-being.
- Keeping a healthy balance between rest and activity by having some exercise every day if you can and by pacing activities throughout the day.
- Identifying anything that is stressful or worrying and allo-
  cating a specific time for problem-solving. It can help to write
  down your concerns.
- Engaging in at least one pleasant activity every day.
- At the end of each day, thinking about three things that you
  found pleasant and writing them down.
- Being aware of unhelpful thinking and considering a calmer
  approach.

  Just remembering which nice things I'd done each day
  helped me cope with what otherwise could have been
  quite a low period.

Less helpful strategies

- Being very busy so that you become exhausted and end up
  sleeping during the day and/or being wakeful at night.
- Keeping problems to yourself and having worries at the back
  of your mind most of the time.

- Not making time for yourself, e.g. for exercise, relaxation or pleasant activities.
- Avoiding certain people or activities.
- Engaging with unhelpful 'catastrophic' thinking.

Which of the helpful and less helpful strategies listed here do you use regularly? If you find you use more of the unhelpful coping methods, give yourself some time to think about how you could change this. Simply trying out some of the strategies in the first list may be enough to help you shift to more positive ways of looking after yourself.

> [I've stopped] getting so uptight about silly things when I've got enough going on in my own life. So now I pick and choose. I'm not going to be sucked into this 'You've got to be here for this, you've got to be here for that . . . we need you for the next thing' scenario.

> I need to do it [the breathing] if I'm getting a lot of hassle at work. As soon as your stress levels go up, [the flushes] come unbelievably. So that's when you think, 'Right, OK'. And that's when I'll shut my door, open my window, stick my fan on and breathe.

Stress and healthy lifestyle: my personal goals

We would like you to think of at least one personal goal that would help you reduce your general level of stress and/or improve well-being. Goals should be simple, specific and achievable. Imagine how you will put your plan into action over the next week – which means considering when, where and how often you will carry out your chosen behaviour. You could, for example, plan to go for a 30-minute walk in a park at lunchtime (between 12:30 and 1:00 p.m.) on Monday, Wednesday and Friday or spend some time in the garden/reading the paper/ having an hour to yourself every evening. Here are some examples from women we have worked with:

> I started to put diary time in for my swimming. Rather than saying, 'oh, I'll try to go swimming on x days this week', I actually started to write down Monday, Wednesday, Friday or whatever. It would be as important to put that in my diary as it would be to have a meeting or something.

> My boss is an absolute terror for wanting things when I'm just about to walk out of the door. But I've had to set

boundaries with him. It's very important for me to get away on time two evenings a week so that I can go to the gym and do the classes that I want to do. That's my time. So I come in earlier, and he knows that. But I have to set those boundaries with him.

I've been literally making about one change a week. . . . I would set myself a target, for example, this week I'm going to get my hair cut, this week I'm going to replace my mattress, and each time I achieved one it's like 'hey, that feels good'.

Taking breaks . . . I'm the only one in the reception area so I'm really, really busy, and it's like sometimes you don't have coffee, you don't have lunch, but allowing yourself to have breaks and be kind to yourself, it really had an impact.

I felt it's important to be consistent to keep doing whatever you can do and that was one of my objectives; my swimming lesson is at nine o'clock on Sunday morning and everyone likes to be in bed [but] I have got up at eight o'clock and gone for my swimming class.

My Stress Goals:

1 . . . .

When?

Where?

How often and how long?

2 . . . .

When?

Where?

How often and how long?

3 You may also have found ways to change stressful thoughts about a situation that is currently stressing you out (or you may practise noticing your inner voice in stressful situations as homework):

Situation:

Stressful thought:

Calmer thought:

Week 1 Homework

- Record hot flushes and night sweats in daily diary.
- Practise relaxation every day using the audio instructions (www.routledge.com/9780367853037), (record practice in diary with an 'X').
- Be aware of hot flush triggers and make a note of them in the daily diary.
- Plan two or three goals for reducing stress and try generally to adopt helpful rather than unhelpful strategies for dealing with stress.

Table 4.1 Hot flush diary, Week 1 Date:

	Monday	Tuesday	Wednesday	Thursday	Friday	Saturday	Sunday
1–6 a.m.							
6–9 a.m.							
9–12 a.m.							
12–2 p.m.							
2–4 p.m.							
4–6 p.m.							
6–8 p.m.							
8–10 p.m.							
10–12 p.m.							

Hot Flushes: Place a √ in the box. Relaxation: Place an X in the correct box.

Night Sweats: Place an o in the box.

Precipitants or activities associated with symptoms:

Printable copies of the diaries in this book are available to download; visit the 'eResources' site: www.routledge.com/9780367853037.

5

Week 2

Managing hot flushes

Managing hot flushes: overview

- Practise relaxation every day, continue stress-reducing goals (you may want to add another this week) and plan your time carefully to avoid rushing.
- Look at your diary and see whether there are any hot flush triggers that you can modify, e.g. too much coffee, rushing to work.
- Check your thoughts – replace negative, 'catastrophizing' thoughts with calming ones.
- At the onset of a flush, let your shoulders relax, breathe slowly from your stomach and concentrate on your breathing – let the flush flow over you as you relax.
- Cool down with sips of water and wear layers but try not to rush out of social situations or avoid doing things that you would usually enjoy.

Understanding hot flushes: a cognitive behavioural approach

This week we are looking at how thoughts and behaviour affect hot flushes.

Managing hot flushes: thoughts and beliefs

As we learned in the stress section, our thoughts can influence the way we feel and behave in certain situations. These thoughts are automatic in that they go through our minds without us really paying attention to them. They reflect ideas or opinions that we have taken on board from a variety of influential sources, such as friends, family or the media. These can have a big impact on how we feel about the flushes and how well we feel able to cope with them.

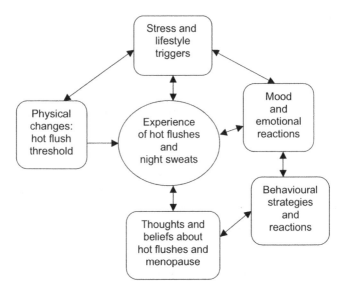

Figure 5.1 Cognitive behavioural model for hot flushes and night sweats

Source: Adapted and reproduced with kind permission from Hunter (2003)

> If I get hot and uncomfortable, I don't suddenly go, 'phew, it's terrible'. I just slowly continue talking and if I get really hot, I just take my cardigan off.

As we described in Chapter 1, menopause has been associated with many negatives in the past (including ageing, ill health and risk of disease). The uncertainty about the menopause, not to mention the value placed on youth and beauty in Western cultures, can make middle-aged and older women actually feel miserable – but this is a stereotype that we can challenge. Look around at the 50-year-olds that you know – there may be a lot going on in their lives, but they rarely match the media's negative stereotype of the 'menopausal woman'.

Now look back at your thoughts about the menopause on page 78. Are these more negative than they need to be?

Negative, stereotypical beliefs about menopause can have a significant influence on how women respond to hot flushes in terms of how they think, feel and behave. If you have particularly negative thoughts during a hot flush, they may conjure up negative emotions and behaviours that can make the experience of the hot flush even worse. So instead of just dealing with the uncomfortable physical sensations of the hot flush, you may also feel embarrassed, ashamed, overwhelmed or exasperated. As with all stressful situations, this can then lead to a vicious cycle.

It's about how I was thinking about it. Why is it so awful? Why is it embarrassing? And we actually looked then at my mum's experience of the menopause. For my mum, it was the worst period of her life – I always thought of it as a bad experience. So, actually recognizing where my thinking was coming from, I still don't like it any better but I am accepting it more as a natural process.

Notice your thoughts when you have a hot flush and write them down:

. . . .
. . . .
. . . .
. . . .
. . . .

Just as we found with the stress-reducing strategies, becoming more aware of our thinking during a hot flush can help to reduce the negative emotions that often accompany it.

Understanding the vicious cycle around hot flushes

Fill in the boxes in Figure 5.2 and think about what your vicious cycle may 'look like' when it comes to hot flushes. It is helpful to think about a specific situation that you find particularly difficult when you have a hot flush.

Situation I find most stressful when having a hot flush (e.g. other people seeing me, feeling out of control or helpless):

. . . .
. . . .
. . . .
. . . .

Now look at the thoughts box in Figure 5.2. If you have difficulty identifying thoughts, consider whether any of the following common examples are true for you.

• Everyone will notice – what will they think?
• Not again!
• These will never end!
• I can't do anything about these!

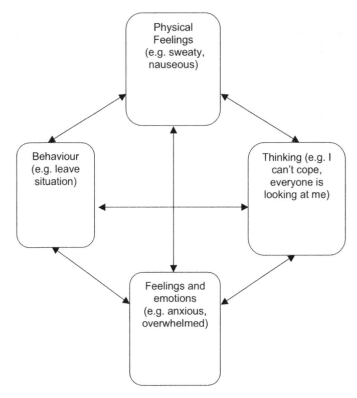

Figure 5.2 Cognitive behavioural 'hot cross bun' model for hot flushes and night sweats

A printable copy of this figure is available to download; visit the 'eResources' site: www.routledge.com/9780367853037

Although there are variations between women, there is evidence to suggest that women have two main types of concerns and feelings during a hot flush (Rendall *et al.* 2008):

1 Concerns about appearance and what others might think, if the flush happens in a social situation. These thoughts can lead to feelings of embarrassment and shame.
2 Concerns about not being able to do anything about the hot flushes, leading to feelings of exasperation, being overwhelmed or out of control.

You may experience one of these more than the other or experience both equally – everybody is different. By looking at these concerns or types of thoughts, you can develop ways of reducing negative reactions to a hot flush. This will help you to feel more in control, and you'll be better able to cope.

Box 5.1

Jane identified that her most problematic hot flushes occurred during handover meetings at the end of a shift at work and when tending to patients. She worried that she looked incompetent in front of others (staff and patients) and felt frustrated about her inability to control the flushes when they occurred – typically, when she was presenting important information to another team. She would lose her concentration and become increasingly flustered as the flush intensified.

Understanding and managing hot flushes in social situations

Women often find social situations particularly difficult during a hot flush and may feel embarrassed about their flushes being visible to, and noticed by, others. This concern can lead to a number of psychological processes, which can increase self-consciousness and embarrassment:

- Viewing yourself through the eyes of others. Instead of focusing attention on the situation, you focus it on yourself – putting yourself in the spotlight – and start to wonder and imagine what everybody else can see. Typical thoughts may be 'Everyone has noticed. What will they think of me?' These are similar to the catastrophic thoughts introduced in Week 1.
- Exaggerated image of yourself. You are likely to base this judgement about your appearance on what you feel like emotionally, so it's all too easy to conclude that you look very hot, red and sweaty. Typical thoughts may be, 'I look ridiculous/unattractive/like I'm having a heart attack'. Often your image of what you look like will be much worse than what people can actually see.
- Increased self-consciousness. These thoughts then lead to more feelings of self-consciousness and embarrassment,

which make the flush even more intense (physical consequences). Because your own attention is focused on yourself, it may start to feel as if everybody else's attention is also on you. In fact, others may not have even noticed the hot flush or are concentrating on other things within the situation.

Research suggests that levels of embarrassment during a public hot flush are associated with how much women are affected by negative stereotypes or beliefs about menopause (Rendall *et al*. 2008). Looking back to page 78, you may have listed some of these too. If so, it is likely that during a hot flush, your embarrassment may be influenced by your awareness of negative images of menopause, which are activated. Other people may (or may not) notice that you are a bit red in the face, but you may feel as though you're wearing red flashing lights, indicating to all that you're going through the menopause.

There are, however, a number of strategies which may help you to manage hot flushes in social situations by reducing feelings of embarrassment. As with paced breathing, you will need to practise these as they involve changing habits of thinking and behaviour in a given situation. In our previous work with women, we have found that when they started to question their thoughts and assumptions about social situations, they were able to change their thinking in the situation, which resulted in them feeling and coping better.

Managing social situations

Many women feel particularly self-conscious during a hot flush as they feel it is a visible sign of their menopause to others. However, people do not necessarily identify hot flush symptoms as being due to menopause and do not have critical or negative reactions towards a woman experiencing them. Looking at the way other people perceive these symptoms and understanding their reactions to them may help you to challenge your views about what others may think if you have a hot flush. This can then help to reduce your anxiety about this happening to you in public.

Even when I'm having a hot flush, I accept that I'm having a hot flush, and if anyone passes a comment I'll acknowledge that I am having a hot flush. And that, mentally, has really reduced my anxiety and I feel more accepting and calmer about it.

What do other people really think about hot flushes?

We conducted a study to answer this question (Smith *et al.* 2011). We asked 290 men and women aged between 25 and 45 for their views and reactions if they saw a 50-year-old woman at work experiencing hot flush symptoms. Without mentioning menopause or hot flushes, they were asked to identify possible causes of redness and sweating. The aim was to see whether they identified the symptoms as a menopausal hot flush and whether this gave rise to negative reactions. The answers are quite illuminating.

As you can see in Box 5.2, over half of those asked thought that the woman's face could be red due to another cause, such as feeling stressed or rather embarrassed. A hormonal cause or menopause was mentioned by roughly 40 per cent, with the majority simply suggesting it was due to 'hormones' or 'hot flush'; women were more likely to consider this a possible cause – only 20 per cent of men linked sweating with hot flushes. One third suggested a minor health problem, such as coming down with a cold. As you can see, people gave a wide variety of reasons and did not all immediately assume menopause. These included physical exertion such as exercise or running up the stairs as the lift had broken, the room being hot or the woman herself being a bit too hot.

Box 5.2

Reasons why the woman may have a red face

Possible reasons:	% men and women:
Emotional cause	52
Hormones or menopause	42
Health problem	35
Warm body temperature	30
Physical exertion	23
Warm environment	21
Skin appearance	18
Food or drink	12

How would you feel about her in the situation?

Feelings:	% men and women:
Empathy, understanding	57
No emotional reaction	25
Consider cause	12
Uncomfortable	10
Consider how to respond helpfully	10
Be led by woman's response	9
Consider how woman may feel	7
Curious about cause	5

The second question – how would you feel about her in this situation? – was included to see whether people really did have the negative reactions that women often assume they do. Almost 60 per cent said that they would feel empathy towards the woman, with 25 per cent feeling neutral. Only 10 per cent said that they felt uncomfortable, but this was because they felt that they were unable to do anything particularly helpful. Importantly, there were no negative reactions towards her, and often people were considering how the woman may be feeling and how they might be able to respond constructively.

My thinking has changed because I know . . . you think people are looking at you and now I've come to accept that they're probably not: it's probably the way you see yourself and so on.

Thinking and behavioural strategies in social situations

So thinking back to common worries in social situations (e.g. 'Everybody has noticed – they may think badly of me'), it may be helpful to remember this survey the next time you have a hot flush in a social situation. Remember, the survey asked about responses to a *severe* hot flush, and it may be that others don't even notice mild or moderate hot flushes, even if you feel as though they do. You can also help yourself by:

- Shifting your focus away from yourself and how you may look and onto breathing through the flush, if the situation allows it.

- If that isn't possible, take a deep breath in, relax your shoulders and then shift your focus of attention away from yourself and onto whatever task you were doing. This takes practice but, over time, can help women feel less self-conscious and anxious. It can also help the flush to pass more quickly.
- Remember that other people are often so preoccupied with their own concerns, daily activities and their view of a given situation that they are unlikely to pay close attention to your hot flush. For example, if you are in a meeting at work and have a flush, even if people *do* notice, they are unlikely to focus on your flush for long. Feeling self-conscious often leads us to assume that other people are as aware of the flush as we are when it happens. But just think about what else people are likely to be thinking about during a meeting at work or in a social situation. For example:

  - the subject of the meeting;
  - whether they have something worthwhile to contribute;
  - what they have to do afterwards;
  - their own issues and worries; or
  - what they are having for dinner that evening.

  As we can see, while anxious thinking may lead you to assume that everyone is 100 per cent focused on your hot flush, once you consider objectively everything else that is going on in the situation, you'll realize that the flush is actually a very small part of that.
- Support yourself by changing the self-critical thoughts you wrote down in the section on your vicious cycle into self-supportive thoughts using the questions from the previous chapter.
- Would you criticize a friend's appearance in the same way in a similar situation or be more supportive towards her? What would you say to her to help her through the situation? Try writing down alternative, more constructive thoughts in response to the hot flush:

  . . . .
  . . . .
  . . . .

  They may not notice, they won't care if they do, or they may feel concerned.
- Make a light-hearted comment or joke if you feel able to – women are often surprised at the positive responses

they get from other people. Remember that in our survey findings, people did not respond negatively and generally wanted to help. We found that women in our research who used this strategy were surprised by the positive responses that people had given them, such as offering to open a window, saying something supportive or empathic or disclosing that they themselves (or their wife in the case of male colleagues) were experiencing hot flushes. It also helped women to know that others didn't really pay attention to their hot flushes as much as they had assumed. However, if the prospect of doing this is daunting or you do not feel it would be appropriate to comment in a specific situation, then don't worry – the aim is to find a strategy that works for *you*.

Here are some comments from women who have used the self-help guide:

> It makes you realize that actually people aren't noticing it as much as you think. . . . In fact, one of the days I was filling in my hot flush diary and I was having a dreadful one and the woman next to me said, 'what's that you're doing?' and I told her. And she said, 'well, actually I'd never noticed you having one' . . . so I was sitting right next to her and she had no idea that I was having one.

> I always used to say I had to explain when I was having a hot flush – 'oh, I'm having a hot flush' – and I now don't bother. . . . I used to get in a do-dah and start flapping my clothes around and things like that . . . feeling I had to explain myself. But I don't have to explain myself if I am a 56-year-old woman and 56-year-old women have hot flushes so it's enabled me to shift my attitude.

Understanding frustration and anxiety with hot flushes

Beyond social situations, many women also report feeling frustrated, annoyed or overwhelmed by their hot flushes generally. This is the other common type of emotional response to hot flushes and happens because we feel unable to control them. Look back to the thoughts box on page 112. You may notice the following thoughts and emotions:

Thoughts	Emotions
Not another one!	Irritated, exasperated, overwhelmed
I can't cope!	Overwhelmed, anxious
This will never end!	Overwhelmed, frustrated, hopeless
These are out of control!	Anxious, helpless, overwhelmed

These thoughts tend to arise in a number of situations, such as having a series of hot flushes in close succession, having flushes when you are relaxing on the sofa watching TV and there is seemingly no trigger or having a flush at a really inconvenient time. While these thoughts are understandable, they can lead to the negative emotions outlined in the table. And when you are feeling exasperated, irritated or overwhelmed, the physical response that arises from these emotions can intensify the hot flush sensations, feeding back into the vicious cycle once more.

When having a hot flush, women often focus on the flush and the attendant physical sensations, but research has shown that doing so can actually intensify these sensations. You can test this out yourself in the task that follows.

Body focus task

1 Pick a part of your body to focus on. This could be your hand, your leg, your knee or your head.
2 Time yourself for two to three minutes, and during this time focus your attention on this part of the body only.
3 In particular, look out for physical sensations or any details that you have not noticed before. Focus your attention fully on any sensations.

What did you notice? Often people report that they notice their pulse or tingling or warmth in the body part. In general people tend to become aware of small sensations that they would not normally pick up on had their attention not been focused on that part of the body. The more they focus, the more they feel physical sensations. It is clear, then, that attention can intensify physical sensations, which again highlights the importance of focusing attention elsewhere during a flush, such as on breathing.

Managing frustrating or overwhelming hot flushes

There are a number of strategies that you can try out to help you manage these types of hot flushes. They involve changing your thinking and behaviour and will therefore take practice. But by removing the negative thinking and emotional response to a flush, you can focus on dealing with the flush itself rather than also having to manage the additional negative emotional reactions which will intensify it further.

> It is mostly the breathing and relaxation, and thinking, 'just let it wash over you and try to relax' [deep, calm, soothing voice]. If I'm cooking or something like that, I'll just stop for a moment.

If you look at the thoughts in the table on page 119, you may notice certain common themes that arise; the thoughts are particularly negative and rule out any possibility of coping from the outset. This is similar to anxious thinking in stressful situations and focusing on the worst possible aspect of the situation. During these flushes, you may forget milder flushes you have actually coped with well or which didn't cause too much disruption. Instead you concentrate all of your attention and negative feelings about hot flushes into this single flush.

The aim is to develop a higher tolerance of the discomfort by choosing to respond differently to it. As we have learned, this won't happen overnight, but persevere. Instead of engaging with the thoughts and emotions of frustration or irritability that intensify the flush and allow it to take over, respond calmly. This may mean taking a deep breath in, relaxing your shoulders and breathing through your flush. Or it may be about changing the negative message you give yourself during a hot flush to a positive self-supportive one. So instead of thinking 'Here we go again!' or 'Not another one!' reassure yourself by thinking 'This will pass soon' or 'Let's see how well I can cope with this one'. Some women report that with practice, adopting a calm response seems to help the flush pass more quickly or makes it feel less severe.

> I don't allow it to bother me. Because I think to myself . . . before it seemed like they last forever and you are getting so many, whereas now it's like they don't last very long. If you had eight in a 24-hour period and they each lasted one or two minutes, what's that in a day?

You may find this tricky at first – thinking and emotional responses are habits that develop over time and become automatic – but take a step back and then actively choose to respond differently. Some women find that if they practise this every time they have a hot flush, it can help to reduce the overall impact that hot flushes have on their day-to-day lives.

> I'm probably still having them but they're not affecting me as such. I'm just carrying on. I just think, 'oh, I'm hot at the moment but it's not a problem'. Because if you think about it you make it into more of a problem, and get hotter still, and more irritated by it.

Other things you can do generally to enhance control are:

- Use paced breathing at the onset of a flush and focus your attention on that instead of the flush. Remember that focusing on the flush itself and monitoring how it develops might actually intensify the physical feelings.
- Modify any triggers you have identified by making general lifestyle changes e.g. reducing alcohol, tea or coffee or avoiding overly spicy foods.
- Plan ahead by wearing light layers that you can remove easily or by having something to distract you if you are entering a situation that typically triggers flushes (e.g. a book for a busy train journey).
- Try to develop an attitude of calm acceptance. Previous research has shown that women who accepted their flushes were significantly less likely to report they had an adverse impact on their day-to-day life.

> I think it was the thing of thinking about it from a different point of view. It's going to happen. You can't stop it. So deal with it. That was a good thing, you know. It made me stop and think.

> Obviously, it's not a thing that you ignore because you can't, at least when they are at the level that they are at for me. I can't ignore them. . . . On the whole, I don't think negatively. If it starts coming and I'm on the train, then I'll read or look out of the window.

If you are finding it difficult to replace unhelpful thinking with neutral or more positive thoughts, here are some responses that women found helpful:

If I was with people I didn't know, I used to think 'well, perhaps they're thinking whatever's the matter with that woman?', particularly men. But I just don't worry about it as much anymore. And if they [flushes] happen I think 'well, it's only going to last a few seconds. I'm not going to collapse'. I mean a flush is not going to last like a cold or flu or sickness that goes on for a day or something like that. That was one thing . . . that this is going to pass very quickly, as soon as I calm myself down . . . it'll be just gone or whatever, you know? It happens to everyone. . . . It's just the life stage I'm at.

Box 5.3

Managing hot flushes: thoughts and beliefs

Notice your thoughts when you have a hot flush: overly negative thoughts can make you feel worse. Try to substitute these for more neutral or helpful thoughts:

Unhelpful thoughts	Helpful thoughts
Oh no, I can't cope.	Let's see how well I can deal with this one.
Everyone's looking at me.	I will notice my flush more than other people will.
I am out of control.	There are things I can do to help control hot flushes.
Hot flushes are bad for my health.	There's no evidence that this is the case – most women have them.
I am ashamed when I have hot flushes.	Hot flushes are part of life.
They will go on forever.	They will gradually reduce over time.
I don't want people to know that I'm going through the menopause.	Menopause is a normal part of life and I shouldn't be ashamed of it.

What would *you* think about someone else with hot flushes?

. . . .
. . . .

Thoughts and breathing

When we begin to see that we have control over our thoughts and realize that they are not reality or facts, we can begin to have more control over our feelings and reactions. By becoming aware of what we are thinking and how we are feeling, we can observe the link between the two and how they interact with our behaviours and bodily symptoms. As noted earlier, adopting a calmer and more supportive thinking response to a hot flush may help you feel less anxious or exasperated by them, and it's very likely that they will feel less intense as a result.

When you are using the paced breathing at the onset of a flush, it may be difficult to keep your attention on the breathing. This is quite normal – just gently refocus on your breathing. Rather than trying to challenge your thoughts during a flush, it is better to simply accept they are there and then spend a few moments refocusing on your breath, consciously relaxing your body . . . and when you have a flush, letting it flow over you. Try to develop an accepting attitude, and don't fight against the flush but instead breathe through it. You can use a calm thought automatically with the breathing if that is helpful, such as 'calm breathing'. In this way you will be able to stop struggling with your thoughts or fighting them and simply allow them to happen, before calmly refocusing your attention on your breathing.

> Before, if I was watching the TV at home and [a flush] would come, I'd reach for the fan, I'd get up and walk around instead of just sitting and letting it go. Now I can distract myself. I concentrate really hard on what's being said on the radio or on the television, or look at a book and just think 'it'll go, it'll go' and then I think 'oh, where's it gone?'. And it's gone. . . . I don't think about the flush. I don't think, 'oh my goodness, am I getting wet? Have I got to wipe myself? Do I need to go and find a cold room?' I don't think of any of those things.

In time you may become more aware of the positive effects of taking a calmer approach to thinking during a hot flush, and you can use the breathing exercise as a pause during which you can think and gather yourself. So breathing can be used in relaxation practice, when you have a flush and also at regular times during the day.

> I found one day I was in one of the big stores at the checkout and I was in a terrible state. And I did the breathing and I started saying, 'This is going to pass, just do the breathing' . . . and it passed and I got through. . . . So the breathing enabled me to give my brain the message that you're not going to pass out, that's not going to happen, and you're going to get through.

> I realized that actually my hot flushes tended to last for only five minutes, and could use that . . . so when I got a hot flush I could tell myself 'oh, this is only going to last a few minutes' and try to calm myself down if at all possible.

Thoughts and breathing during hot flushes and stress

As we mentioned in Week 1, breathing can be helpful during stressful situations as well as at the onset of a flush. Most of the time we don't even notice our breathing, but it can tell us a lot about how we are feeling or thinking. Deep, slow breaths may indicate feelings of relaxation, while short, quick breaths or holding the breath too long, feeling tight in the chest and shallow breathing all point to rising stress levels. Becoming aware of your breathing will, with practice, help you manage hot flushes and can help to reduce your general stress levels. It is helpful to start that practice during everyday, low-pressure situations.

> I discovered [that] if I concentrate on my breathing, it makes me think about the hot flush less once I get it. Initially it makes you think about it more. You think 'oh no, I'm having a hot flush, I have got to do breathing' but as it goes on, you just start to breathe in and you don't really notice your hot flush so much.

For example, you're waiting in a queue, and the person in front is really slow. It's easy to become irritated or impatient, but instead quietly draw yourself together and acknowledge that you're irritated – e.g. 'I feel really annoyed', or 'I can feel my frustration levels rising'. Follow that with becoming aware of your breath as it flows in and out of your body. It can help to be quite conscious of the process and say to yourself: 'Breathing in, stomach expanding. Breathing out, stomach softening' or something similar. Feel the body 'letting go' with each outward breath. Coming back to our scenario, once you have followed the breath for a minute or so, the situation may well have resolved itself, and you'll have had the pleasure of a few minutes of calming breath. Or if not, you have at least created space in your mind to decide how to react. This is similar to choosing to react in a calm way to hot flushes; you can either go with your anger and frustration or acknowledge those feelings and then focus on breathing until you feel calmer, and the symptoms pass.

> Well, I do some deep breathing when I really get angered at work. . . . [S]ome colleagues can get you really, really frustrated, you know, so I find it helps to take a big breath.

You could also imagine you are having a hot flush and practise:

RELAX → SLOWBREATHING → CALMING THOUGHTS

> You have to alter your mind-set. If you leave that where it is, then the paced breathing is not going to do anything. If you're still stressing out and thinking, 'This is awful; I hate it', then the paced breathing is not going to work because you're getting more and more stressed.

Behavioural reactions to hot flushes

Although there is never a good time to experience a hot flush, some situations may be worse than others, e.g. at work, in a social situation. Therefore, it is useful to think about what you do when you have flushes and what might help.

What do you tend to do when you have a hot flush? (behaviour)

. . . .
. . . .

Leaving the room or avoiding situations may help in the short term, but in the long term, it can make things worse as you may retreat into yourself and become increasingly anxious about attending work or personal events. You are also giving yourself the message that you can't cope. It is generally better, then, to stay in a given situation when you have a hot flush so that you learn that you can cope. This can also help to make the hot flush less threatening and reduce the impact it has on your life in general.

Practical behaviours that can help

- Using paced breathing and relaxation followed by refocusing your attention on your surroundings.
- Accepting the flushes rather than fighting them.
- Pacing your activities so that you don't have to rush.
- Pausing to decide how to react or what strategy to use in a situation.
- Taking your time to adjust if you move from a cold to a hotter room.
- Wearing light layers which can be easily removed.
- Using humour or acknowledging it by commenting about it to others if you feel comfortable doing this.
- Trying not to avoid doing things because of hot flushes.

Deep breath in and relax shoulders → Let the flush flow over you → Paced breathing

Once relaxed, refocus your attention on your surroundings and continue with your day.

> At first it was the paced breathing and the relaxation. I'd get into it. Now I don't really even need to think about that. It just happens. It's become a pattern – a way of behaving. I don't even think, 'oh God, I've got to do my paced breathing and my relaxation'. It just happens.

> Just all of a sudden once it clicked, and you started to understand it, and you found yourself doing the breathing, and you notice they [the flushes] weren't as long . . . and then you thought 'well, that's not too bad actually'.

Box 5.4

After reading through the information in the book, Jane decided to change her behavioural response to hot flushes. Instead of going with anxious worries that others may think she was incompetent, she planned to focus on breathing and telling herself to keep calm. Jane found it difficult to directly challenge her perception of being out of control but found the survey helped her to remember that she was making assumptions about others' reactions to her. The following week during a meeting with staff, Jane experienced a huge hot flush and lost her train of thought. Instead of panicking, she asked for a brief moment to gather her thoughts and asked the staff to come back to her in a few minutes. The handover continued, and Jane took this time to breathe and remind herself to keep calm and focus on the information that she needed to communicate. The meeting then returned to her, and she was able to continue in a calmer way. Jane was struck by how everyone's attention was on the content of the discussion, rather than on her efforts to compose herself, and found this a positive and helpful experience, which improved her confidence. It helped her to start to reconsider her beliefs about hot flushes that led to her feeling out of control.

Week 2 Homework

- Fill in the Hot Flush Rating Scale for Week 2 and record hot flushes and night sweats in the Weekly Diary.
- Think about ways of reducing triggers: for example, cutting down on hot drinks or rushing about less. Everyone is different, so you will need to experiment to find out what works best for you.
- Continue your relaxation practice using the relaxation and breathing recording every day if you can (record relaxation practice in diary with an X) and breathe slowly at the onset of a hot flush, letting the flush flow over you.
- Be aware of your thinking about your flushes and try to adopt more helpful thoughts.
- If your sleep is affected by night sweats, please monitor your sleep pattern over the next week using the sleep diary at the end of this section. This will provide useful information for Week 3.
- Deal with hot flushes and stress using the following sequence:

RELAX → SLOW BREATHING → CALMING THOUGHTS

Sleep diary

The sleep diary is designed to help you keep a record of your sleep experiences. Please complete one column of the diary each morning, soon after you wake up. Take a few minutes to do this, trying to be as accurate as you can. However, remember that it is your *best estimate* that we are looking for: we don't want you to get into the habit of clockwatching at night or to become overly preoccupied by sleep. To calculate how long you slept (8):

1 Add rows 4 (total time to get to sleep) to the total time awake in question 5 to get the total awake time during the night.
2 Then subtract that amount from row 3 (time in bed) to get a reasonably accurate estimate of your total sleep time.

Table 5.1 Sleep diary

	Mon	Tues	Wed	Thurs	Fri	Sat	Sun	Example
1. What time did you get up out of bed this morning?								*6:15 a.m.*
2. What time did you go to bed last night? (turned the light out)								*11:00 p.m.*
3. How many hours between going to bed and getting up? (time in bed)								*7 hrs 15mins*
4. How long did it take you to fall asleep (hrs)?								*30mins*
5. How many times did you wake up during the night?								*4*
6. How many of these times were due to having a night sweat?								*3*
7. How much time you were awake during the night? (i.e. add **4** to the total time awake from when awake in **5**)								*30mins + 1hr 15mins*
8. About how long did you sleep altogether (hrs)? (**3**–**7**) (Total sleep time)								*5hrs 30mins*

Printable copies of the diaries in this book are available to download, visit the 'eResources' site www.routledge.com/9780367853037

Table 5.2 Hot flush diary, Week 2 Date:

	Monday	Tuesday	Wednesday	Thursday	Friday	Saturday	Sunday
1–6 a.m.							
6–9 a.m.							
9–12 a.m.							
12–2 p.m.							
2–4 p.m.							
4–6 p.m.							
6–8 p.m.							
8–10 p.m.							
10–12 p.m.							

Printable copies of the diaries in this book are available to download; visit the 'eResources' site: www.routledge.com/9780367853037

Week 3

Managing sleep and night sweats

Sleep and night sweats

This week we are going to look at night sweats and sleep. By now we hope you are feeling more at ease with the relaxation exercises, have incorporated some helpful strategies and pleasant activities into your day-to-day life and have maybe started to challenge some of your thoughts about menopause and hot flushes. This week we will turn our attention to applying CBT to night sweats and sleep. Sometimes just a few small changes to our evening routine can make a big difference to how well we rest through the night. Night sweats do wake women up at night, and the aim here is to help you get into an automatic routine of dealing with them calmly. If you have disturbed sleep, you can use the information in this section to improve your sleep routines and to help you to get back to sleep.

Box 6.1

Jane's sleep had improved slightly since she had started managing stress at work, but her sleep was still interrupted by night sweats at times. She found it difficult to get back to sleep and would lie awake worrying about how she'd get through the next day. Her anxious thoughts led her to anticipate that she'd struggle, and, as a result, she often cancelled social activities planned for the next evening so that she could catch up on sleep. However, she still found it difficult to sleep the following night despite being exhausted.

In this section, we'll look at some of the steps you can take to train your body and mind to have a reasonable night's sleep, including regular relaxation practice. First, we will run through some information about sleep from research evidence. Then we will look at habits, lifestyle influences and bedroom environment before finally focusing on sleep behaviours, worrying thoughts and your feelings and beliefs about sleep. Becoming aware of what is happening before going to bed – and while you're there – can help you work out what changes you need to make to help yourself. Have a good look at your sleep diary – this will be useful in the following section.

Understanding sleep

- Each night we go through approximately four to five sleep cycles, which include REM (rapid eye movement) and non-REM sleep. Each cycle lasts for between 90 and 110 minutes (see Figure 6.1). Each complete sleep cycle is one of the peaks and troughs in the figure.
- REM sleep comes and goes throughout the night, making up about one fifth of our sleep time. During REM, our brains are very active, and our bodies are relaxed. We dream and our eyes move around quickly.
- Non-REM sleep includes the rest of our sleep and occurs in four stages. Stages one and two are lighter stages of sleep,

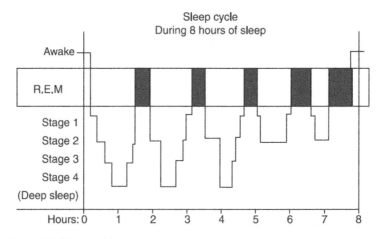

Figure 6.1 Stages of sleep

Source: http://ygraph.com/chart/2076

during which we can be easily woken. Stages three and four are deeper levels of restorative 'slow wave' sleep, which tend to occur more during the first half of the night. We then spend the rest of the night alternating between REM and stage two sleep. As we go into deeper stages of sleep, our bodies naturally cool, our blood pressure drops and our bodies release hormones and transmitters that help to repair wear and tear from the day.

There are a couple of important points to be aware of when looking at the sleep cycle shown in this chapter:

- Sleep is not a simple 'on-off' mechanism like a light switch. It is actually more helpful to think of sleep as a kind of 'dimmer switch'; our brain goes from being fully alert (when we are awake) into different stages of reduced awareness or consciousness. This can have an impact on our perceptions of sleep and how much we have had. There is more about the impact of this on our perception of sleep in the next section.
- Deep restorative sleep (stages three and four) takes place at the beginning of the night. If you have not slept well the night before, your body automatically catches up the next night by entering these stages more quickly – we are biologically programmed to do so. Even if sleep is broken as the night goes on, you are likely to have 'good enough' restorative sleep.
- As the night goes on, your sleep naturally becomes lighter, and as noted earlier, in the second half of the night you alternate between light sleep (stages one and two) and REM sleep. Therefore, you are more likely to notice night sweats when you are in the lighter stages of sleep.
- Periods of waking are normal throughout the night. Whenever people are measured in a sleep laboratory, their readings always indicate a minute or two of waking (as indicated by the two highest peaks on Figure 6.1), but they rarely remember it. You are more likely to remember waking if you are having night sweats or are anxious about something.

How much sleep do we really need?

Although disturbed sleep can be upsetting, we can often manage on a lot less than we think. What we need very much depends on our age. Children need nine to ten hours, but this then reduces as we get older. A normal adult average is six to seven hours per night.

A study examining sleep and health data from over one million people showed that those who slept between six and eight hours per night had better health outcomes than those who consistently slept less than five or more than nine. So while everyone differs, it seems that six to eight hours is optimal and that needing to sleep eight hours or more is a myth (Ferrie *et al.* 2007).

Sleep perceptions

Because sleep is a different state of awareness, our judgements about it are not always accurate. There is evidence that three factors can influence our take on how much sleep we've actually had:

1 Sleep inertia. It is common to still feel 'dazed' or 'half asleep' for up to 30 minutes after waking, but this is the time in which we are most likely to reflect on our night's sleep and decide whether or not we have slept well. Because we still feel a little 'fuzzy', we may conclude that we've slept poorly. We also may assume that the dazed feeling will be with us all day, but actually we will have forgotten about it 30 minutes later once we've had a cup of tea or a shower.
2 Sleep onset. Stages one and two of sleep are a bit of a mystery. It is difficult to measure when exactly we fall asleep, and research has shown that we are most likely to report being awake when a machine that measures sleep shows we were in fact slumbering (Bonnet 1990).
3 Worry. Research has also found that because our minds often race when we worry, 30 minutes of trying to sleep can feel much longer (Borkovec 1982).

Therefore:

- We tend to underestimate how much sleep we get.
- We tend to overestimate the time it takes us to go to sleep.
- If we learn about this tendency to misjudge, we worry less and sleep better.

It may be helpful to remind yourself about this if you feel worried about any sleep disruption.

> Some people say they don't sleep and actually they do. Where I used to live, the man next door used to have a grandfather clock and it used to chime. . . . I'd think, 'if I hear it at midnight and then I don't hear it again till five

o'clock in the morning, then I know that I slept for five hours'. Sometimes you don't realize that you have slept. And you perceive that you've had this terrible night when actually it hasn't been that bad.

Strategies to improve sleep quality and reduce disruption

Over the next few pages we will look at a variety of strategies to help you to cope if your sleep is disrupted by night sweats and/or stress. These involve:

- Getting into better sleeping habits by making minor changes to your sleeping environment and behaviour at bedtime.
- Restricting activities in the bedroom mainly to sleeping in order to help you develop a strong association between bedtime and sleep.
- Using automatic and routine responses when you are woken by night sweats to help you manage nighttime waking calmly.
- Helping you to focus on your daily life regardless of sleep difficulties.
- Managing worries about night sweats and sleep.

On a practical level, the breathing exercises have really helped, especially at night. . . . I just lie there, take the quilt off my chest, which feels to me like it's burning, and I just flip the duvet up and do the breathing exercises for 10 or 20 seconds, and it just goes.

Sleep habits and helpful strategies

In order to develop good sleep habits, it is worth spending some time thinking about lifestyle and environmental factors that might make a difference to your sleep.

Lifestyle factors

Limit caffeine and nicotine

Caffeine and nicotine are stimulants and can affect the amount of time it takes you to fall asleep as well as the amount of time you spend in deep sleep. Avoiding caffeine completely for up to four hours before bedtime is recommended, although research has shown that any caffeine after 2 p.m. can have an impact on your ability to fall asleep in the evening.

Limit alcohol

Although alcohol may help you drop off initially, it reduces sleep quality, and you are likely to wake up early as your body works hard to detoxify your system. It also limits deep restorative sleep, leading to excessive tiredness the next day. So if you are drinking alcohol, it makes sense to leave a few hours between your last drink and going to bed.

Manage diet

Eating a heavy meal before bedtime can also keep you awake, so leave at least three hours between eating and sleep. Include carbohydrates in your evening meal as they help your brain to release sleep-inducing chemicals. A glass of warm milk or a banana can have a similar effect.

Manage exercise

Exercise helps you to fall asleep more quickly and improves sleep quality, but it is best to avoid intense exercise immediately before bedtime as it may keep you awake.

> I can't really drink much alcohol these days. My friends are fine but we are all different. It's difficult because people say 'come on, have a glass of wine'. But really, it's just not worth it for me. I think, 'shall I?' and then I think, 'no, I won't, because really I'd just rather enjoy this food and sleep'.

Environmental factors

Limit noise

Noise can prevent us from falling asleep, so if you have a partner who snores or noisy neighbours, invest in some earplugs.

Manage room temperature

Ideally, your room should be on the cooler side as the body loses heat naturally as you fall asleep. Open the window if possible or invest in a fan. It's also a good idea to avoid big duvets and opt for thinner layers of bedding or clothing that can be adjusted easily.

Improve air quality

A clean bedroom environment improves breathing and sleep.

Improve bed comfort

A comfortable bed can add over 30 minutes to your sleep time compared to an uncomfortable one, so it is worth investing in a good mattress.

Is there anything that you could change to help your sleep habits?

. . . .
. . . .
. . . .
. . . .

I always have cotton sheets, anyway. They're always very cool and I can just stretch my legs out straight and relax and let the sweats flow, so that's good.

If I was ever woken up by a night sweat, I was terrible for checking the time, the clock – so now I don't do it. I usually have my lavender oil nearby, so maybe I'll reach out and just put a little bit on. And then I roll over and I don't even get up for a drink.

I've actually turned the radiator off in my bedroom. It has been nice and cold. My husband does complain but I'll have the window open and my bedroom is icy and actually the colder I make it, the less I'm going to wake up in the night.

So it made me assess things like, I've now got a fan in my bedroom. I don't ever have a winter duvet on anymore.

Sleep scheduling and associating bed with sleep

Look back at your sleep diary and work out how much sleep you usually have. Remember that most people function well on seven hours, so if you go to bed at midnight and get up at 7 a.m., you are probably having enough sleep to manage on. Regular sleep habits are very helpful – you can develop good sleep habits using the following rules of 'sleep scheduling' and associating bed with sleep (Espie 2010).

Sleep scheduling helps regulate your body clock, thereby improving sleep quality. We can fall into irregular habits quite easily – this commonly happens after jet lag, for example – so in a way we have to teach our bodies to relearn 'good sleep practice'. Building the association between bed and sleep means you are more likely to fall asleep quickly when you are in bed! These methods need to be applied regularly and consistently over time to work best; they will not have any effect if done on one night only (Harvey 2002).

Sleep scheduling

Plan the times that you want to sleep and stick to them. For example, getting up at 7 a.m. following a midnight bedtime will give you a total sleep time of seven hours.

Associating bed with sleep

This can be challenging but is worth it if you have poor sleep habits.

- Use your bed only for sleep (and sex, if this applies to you).
- Lie down in bed only when you feel sleepy.
- Keep laptops and TVs out of the bedroom; they promote wakefulness and weaken the link between bed and sleep.
- Don't nap. If you absolutely have to, do so before 3 p.m. and for no longer than one hour.
- Avoid lying in or going to bed early to compensate for a bad night: sticking to set bedtimes and getting up times, regardless of how much sleep you've had, helps your body clock to reset itself. Trying to compensate by going to bed earlier can paradoxically mean that you lie awake for hours and become even more stressed about not sleeping – leading to more frustration and less sleep.
- Keep the bedroom dark, as this will trigger sleepiness.

Use breathing exercises and the relaxation recording if you need help winding down at bedtime. If a night sweat wakes you, cool down and then use breathing to calm your thoughts and return to bed to sleep.

Wind-down routines

Developing a good wind-down routine can be helpful. You should aim to do relaxing activities 60 to 90 minutes before you go to bed. Anything that helps you to switch off from your day and relax – such as having a warm bath or reading – will help prepare your body for going to sleep. You may also want to practise the relaxation exercises.

Learning to relax is like learning a new skill. Like sleep, it involves the 'letting go' principle. As you become more accustomed to it, it can be used as an automatic response whenever you are woken by night sweats.

Before you go to bed, what do you actually do? Maybe if you take tea or coffee again they can set you off and leave you awake tossing and turning. So I changed all that to a milky drink. . . . Even sometimes just having a nice bath with some candles around, so sort of preparing myself.

Managing daytime tiredness

While it is tempting to cancel plans and attempt to rest if you are tired after a bad night, you should still aim to continue with your day as planned. Limiting activities can actually result in increased levels of tiredness as your attention becomes focused on your sleep disruption. Continuing as normal with plans, on the other hand, provides a distraction and can take your mind off feeling tired. If you do feel weary, try pacing your activities rather than cancelling them completely or doing something to energize yourself, such as going for a brief brisk walk in the fresh air. It is also generally more helpful to use relaxation rather than naps to manage tension arising from tiredness.

If I get very tired, I'm getting better at managing that now because I've realized I don't have to go to sleep if I'm tired. I can just relax, breathe, do the relaxation thing, take 10 minutes.

If this sounds unlikely, try doing both (limiting activities versus continuing as normal) on two days when you have missed sleep. Rate your tiredness out of 10 at two-hourly intervals on both days – 10 would be the most tired you have ever been, and 0 would be feeling absolutely alert and fine. Research shows that you are more likely to feel tired on days when you limit your activities than on days when you carry on as planned.

I've had one or two nights where the symptoms have become quite severe again but I've just breathed, relaxed, stuck my fan on, and almost mentally switched off from it. And the realization that even if you have a bad night's sleep, you're going to get through the next day. . . . Don't let it be negative; have a positive view instead, 'I'll be fine'.

Sleep and worrying thoughts

Worrying thoughts are usually distressing and cause us to become restless and agitated. This is especially the case at night when we feel less in control. It is not surprising they keep us awake, as we need to be relaxed to drop off. So rather than engaging with these thoughts, try to deal with them before they result in worry:

- Allow thoughts to come and go, e.g. like a train passing through a station or a river flowing by.
- Focus on your breathing or a pleasant calming image.
- If the thought does take hold (this is more likely if the thoughts consist of fears), substitute more helpful, neutral and realistic thoughts using the questions from the stress section. You may need to do this again in the daytime so that the alternative, calming thoughts are prepared for you (page 97).
- Be firm in telling yourself that you will assign yourself a set 'worry time' the next day (in the daytime) during which you will think specifically about the problem that concerns you. (It may be useful to utilize the problem-solving approach at that time.)

> I was waking up in the middle of the night and going over and over a conversation, 'what could I have said better?' [Instead] 'I'm only going to think about this at 10 o'clock tomorrow' – brilliant!

What sort of things might run through your head if you can't sleep? Write them down here, e.g. 'I'm never going to be able to concentrate at work tomorrow', or 'If I wake up, I'll never get back to sleep'.

. . . .
. . . .
. . . .
. . . .

How did these thoughts make you feel? It is likely that they made you feel anxious, worried or miserable. Rate how strong these feelings were on a scale of 0 to 10 (0 being not at all and 10 being the worst ever!), e.g. 'I won't be able to do anything at work tomorrow!' Anxious, 9/10.

Dealing with worrying thoughts

As we learned earlier, anxious thoughts can lead to the body's stress response (fight or flight). This results in the release of adrenaline, which will make falling asleep less likely. Anxious thoughts also tend to undermine our coping and make the situation worse. However, we can come up with calmer alternatives that will help us feel less fretful, both physically and emotionally.

> I stopped having the clock next to me because I realized that it was a very negative thing to do. I would keep looking and, 'oh no, it's two o'clock; oh no, it's three o'clock', so that would make me feel even worse.

As noted earlier, anxious thoughts tend to be very all or nothing. For example, thoughts such as 'I won't be able to function at all!' or 'I'll feel exhausted all day!' are pretty extreme reactions.

As a result, we focus on the worst possible outcome (catastrophizing) and ignore any middle ground. Think about the last time you missed sleep and how you coped the following day. If these two thoughts were 100 per cent, then you would have been unable to think or do anything at all and would sit near to 0 per cent on the scale! This seems unlikely. You may well have felt tired at points throughout the day or struggled occasionally with concentration, but most likely you managed to do whatever tasks you needed to and felt reasonably all right. Realistically, you're more likely to be somewhere in the middle of this range, functioning 'well enough' – probably around 50 per cent.

Also, even on days when sleep has been fine, we are unlikely to perform at 100 per cent all day long! So instead, try to identify

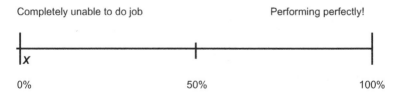

Completely unable to do job   Performing perfectly!

0%   50%   100%

Figure 6.2 Predicting how you will feel and function the next day following disturbed sleep

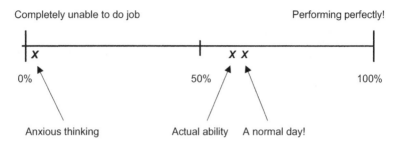

Figure 6.3 How do we actually function the next day following disturbed sleep?

a more helpful perspective based on your previous experience of managing on little sleep. Here are some examples:

I can get on with usual things even if I have had a bad night's sleep.

Sleep problems are not dangerous or bad for me.

I may look a bit tired but will not have aged 10 years overnight!

My helpful thought is:

. . . .
. . . .
. . . .

Now rate your anxiety or worry again on a scale of 0 to 10. Has it reduced?

And also, a little trick that I use and it worked and has stayed working is, 'If I'm not going to sleep, who cares!' and then you're off. Instead of 'I need to go to sleep. I need to go to sleep. I need to go to sleep', I don't do that now.

Strategies to use if night sweats disturb your sleep

Helpful strategies

- Getting on with normal things even if you have not slept well – your body rhythms will see you through the day.
- Recognizing that sleep problems are not dangerous.
- Remembering that most people feel tired as they are waking up.

- Remembering that most people overestimate how much sleep they need.
- Keeping realistic expectations, e.g. everyone will have a poor night's sleep occasionally.
- Recognizing that not feeling completely rested some days is normal, even after a good night's sleep!
- Also recognizing that there are some things within your control. For example, you can keep your sleep schedule regular, cut out negative lifestyle influences from your life and your bedroom area, refrain from napping in the daytime and not spend too much time in bed.

Unhelpful strategies

- Exaggerating the seriousness as this can lead to more worry, e.g. 'I look 10 years older after no sleep last night'.
- Letting your world revolve around sleep.
- Cancelling activities; this will only give you more time to worry about the upcoming night.

I used to have trouble getting off to sleep because I used to lie there thinking 'I'm going to have a terrible night's sleep'. I would worry about what I was going to do if I only got so much sleep. And now, I don't think about it. I go to bed. I read a book.

Summary of sleep advice

- By managing your sleep, you can deal with night sweats in a calmer, more automatic way:

  COOL DOWN → BREATHING → CALM THOUGHTS → RELAX AND RETURN TO BED

- Manage unhelpful environmental and lifestyle factors and maintain a regular sleep pattern:
  - Restrict your time in bed to your average actual sleep time.
  - No napping – use relaxation during the day to manage tiredness or tension arising from missed sleep.
  - Keep your bed mainly for sleep.
- Manage worrying thoughts – about various concerns you may have and/or about sleep:
  - Let the thoughts (as well as the night sweats) flow over you; don't engage with them.

- ○ Use relaxation and paced breathing.
- ○ Try to develop a flexible, more accepting attitude (calming), rather than one of annoyance or exasperation (restlessness).
- ○ Arrange 'worry time' to problem solve during the daytime, for a set period.
- Practise relaxation and breathing to:

  - ○ Reduce overall stress by providing balance to busy lives.
  - ○ Manage hot flushes/night sweats and induce sleepiness when required.
  - ○ Develop a good bedtime wind-down routine.

Responding calmly to night sweats

Your response to night sweats draws on the strategies that you have learned previously in this book. These strategies link anxious thinking and behaviour to anxious physiological responses that will keep you awake longer.

Therefore, the aim when having a night sweat is to try to remain calm using the following strategies:

- Calmly get up and do whatever you need to cool down.
- Practise paced breathing as an automatic response.
- Watch your thoughts while you are doing this. If they have become worried or anxious, remember they are just thoughts rather than facts about the situation. Think back to alternative responses you may have generated on previous pages.
- Once you have cooled off, get back into bed and practise relaxation and paced breathing. Some women find it helpful to have the relaxation recording near the bed so they can switch it on quickly and easily without thinking too much about having woken up.
- Be aware of your thoughts but don't engage with them. Instead, return the focus of your attention to your breathing. This will be easier the more you practise.

Box 6.2

Jane was reassured by reading about the sleep cycle and realised that her body would make sure that she got enough deep sleep the following night even if she woke up a few times. She again used the thinking strategies and identified that her thinking was unhelpful as it caused her even more anxiety, which in turn made it difficult to sleep. Jane recalled all of the occasions when she had gone into work and, although feeling tired, had become distracted in her tasks and had been able to function at a 'good enough' level to get her work done. Therefore, she could see that her predictions about not functioning were not accurate. Jane practised not engaging with these thoughts when they occurred at 3 a.m. and instead focused on paced breathing. She found that this made it more likely that she would fall back to sleep. Jane also tested out keeping arrangements with friends (a good stress reliever) and found that instead of focusing on her tiredness, she could enjoy herself and return home feeling more relaxed, with work in perspective. This helped her to relax at bedtime, and in a few weeks, she was less anxious about night sweats and her sleep quality improved. When woken by a night sweat, she would automatically and calmly cool off and then start the breathing and relax any tense muscles.

When you can't get back to sleep and you're tossing and turning and you end up watching TV or something, that's probably the worst thing you can do. I used to do that. . . . [W]ell I don't need to [now] because I can just get back to sleep. It's not a problem. I wake up, go to the loo, wipe down my chest and forehead, and just get back into bed and go to sleep.

Managing sleep and night sweats: my personal goals

We would like you to think of two goals aimed at improving your sleep pattern. Goals should be simple, specific and achievable. Imagine how you will put your plan into action over the next week – which means when, where and how often you will carry out your chosen behaviour.

1 ....

  ....

When?

Where?

How often and how long?

2 ....

   ....

When?

Where?

How often and how long?

Week 3 Homework

- Keep practising the relaxation and paced breathing exercises.
- Schedule an enjoyable activity every day.
- Review your goals for reducing stress.
- Write down and carry out your goals for sleeping and managing night sweats.
- Continue to use breathing and calming thoughts when you feel stressed and at the onset of a flush.
- Please fill in the Hot Flush Rating Scale and diary for Week 3.

  RELAX → SLOW BREATHING → CALMING THOUGHTS

Table 6.1 Hot flush diary, Week 3 Date:

	Monday	Tuesday	Wednesday	Thursday	Friday	Saturday	Sunday
1–6 a.m.							
6–9 a.m.							
9–12 a.m.							
12–2 p.m.							
2–4 p.m.							
4–6 p.m.							
6–8 p.m.							
8–10 p.m.							
10–12 p.m.							

Printable copies of the diaries in this book are available to download; visit the 'eResources' site: www.routledge.com/9780367853037

7

Week 4

Reviewing and maintaining changes

The menopausal transition: a time to reflect

As well as the physical changes that accompany menopause, many women also experience it as a major life transition involving social role changes, such as children leaving home or increased responsibility for older relatives and often increased responsibility at work. These changes can sometimes be distressing; not only do they bring uncertainty and possible time pressures, but they may also affect how you think about yourself. You may well find yourself reflecting on past events and feeling anxious about what the future holds. These feelings are normal and understandable, though, and often accompany transitional life stages.

Think back over other big life changes you've gone through (for example, adolescence, starting or ending an important relationship, changing jobs or having children) and write down how you felt at the time. People often report a mix of positive feelings, such as hopefulness, and anxiety about the future or uncertainty about the impact of a certain situation on themselves.

Other life changes I have experienced:

. . . .
. . . .
. . . .

Even changes in the past that eventually proved to be positive may have provoked anxiety at the time, but you will have drawn on your resources and managed the change, gradually adapting to it and developing as a person. The same applies to the changes that can accompany menopause. Here, we have summarized some helpful strategies to help you to manage this process. These have been drawn from our previous work with women who faced the same anxieties and uncertainties but who eventually adapted to the physical and psycho-social changes that can occur during midlife.

- Remember this is a normal life stage, and the feelings that accompany it are not uncommon. Be confident that you will navigate through the changes.

  It's part of life. There are thousands of other women going through it.

- Look after yourself – it is especially important to do so during times of change. This will put you in a better position to cope with any challenges. You can do this using the strategies covered in Chapter 4, such as scheduling pleasant activities and pacing your activities. Also take a moment to notice your own positive qualities – it's all too easy to overlook them.

  I think I've become a bit selfish at times and I think, 'actually, this weekend is for me' and I do try to take time to do things for me. The last few weekends I've been busy helping my daughter get back to university. It's been quite stressful and I haven't actually been at home. So I'm actually looking forward to being a bit selfish this weekend and to just having a bit of me-time.

- Be open to new experiences to fill any 'empty' spaces that may arise during this time of transition. Be aware in particular of negative thoughts about ageing (e.g. 'I'm too old to try new things') that limit opportunities. There is no rule book that dictates what people can and can't do. Instead try adopting a 'why not?' attitude.

  I've become a lot more relaxed to myself and [am] understanding the whole element that it's just a phase in your life, you have to just do it, accept it and get on with life.

- Are there any activities you used to enjoy or get a sense of achievement from that you might have given up when job or family priorities took over? If so, can you take them up again now? Perhaps there are classes or activities in your local area that you could take up – a friend could go with you to begin with. We have found that women who pursue activities they are interested in are more likely to feel hopeful and positive about the future.

I do a lot of painting now. I hadn't done it for years, but I started doing that again, and it was that bit of being nice to myself.

I've realised I've been taking more and more on at work without discussing this in my review – to help reduce stress I'm going to talk to my manager and realistically prioritise what needs to be done and what I can delegate or do in a few months time.

I've been getting rid of a load of clothes that didn't fit which was once again a big step for me because in a way it's like putting your past behind you, but at the same time it's a sort of acceptance because you're accepting. . . . I'll move on, and gradually over the course of time maybe even get a few new ones.

In the last couple of weeks I've joined a sports club mainly to go swimming but also to do aqua aerobics. And this is an absolutely massive step for me. I haven't done anything like this since I was at university.

Dealing with menopausal symptoms related to breast cancer treatment

Common reactions to breast cancer and its treatment

A diagnosis of breast cancer can have a huge emotional impact. You may experience mood swings and tearfulness, and it may even impact on your beliefs about yourself. These reactions are all part of the normal adjustment process but can take some time to work through. So accept that you are dealing with a physical and emotional adjustment and make sure you talk to others and take things gradually. Don't feel bad (guilty or self-critical) if you have strong emotions – again, these are part of the adjustment to the situation.

You may feel anxious about the uncertainty you are facing or the possibility of the cancer coming back. In a broader per-spective, life is full of uncertainties, but most of the time we cope by trying to avoid thinking about them. Can you think of an occasion where you have faced uncertainty in the past but coped with it? What did you do to help you cope?

. . . .
. . . .
. . . .

Helpful and unhelpful cognitive and behavioural reactions

While it is completely normal and understandable to feel anxious about breast cancer, as in other situations, overly negative and pessimistic thoughts can make you feel helpless and have a negative impact on your mood. Some reactions – such as body checking and seeking reassurance – might prolong feelings of anxiety. You may also find yourself avoiding day-to-day normal activities, feeling that 'small things' are trivial and not worth bothering with. Trying to maintain some semblance of 'normal' life can be helpful, though, and will help contribute to a positive overall well-being.

Beware of black-and-white thinking, which can often happen when people are under pressure. In this context you might see yourself as either 100 per cent well or 100 per cent unwell. If you view yourself as 100 per cent unwell, you may be inclined to withdraw and reduce your activities in an attempt to protect yourself. However, this may have a negative impact on your mood. Alternatively, when you see yourself as 100 per cent well, you may well go 'full throttle', expecting yourself to do everything that you used to do before your breast cancer diagnosis, and end up exhausted. The danger with this is that you can end up in a 'boom and bust cycle'. It's important to remember that it can take a while for your body to recover from breast cancer treatments: some women report that it can take one to two years before their energy levels return to normal.

What can help?

- Recognise and counter thoughts that are overly negative.
- Encourage self-supportive thinking and give yourself time to adjust.
- Use behavioural strategies such as activity scheduling (scheduling pleasant events) to help to balance out low mood and anxieties and provide distraction. Try not to minimize the importance of 'little things' as they are often extremely important.
- Make use of social support. People will be happy to help, so it's important to acknowledge if help is needed.
- Try to adapt and/or reduce demands on yourself to counter tiredness following your illness – be aware of black-and-white thinking and pace activities to avoid the 'boom and bust' pattern.

- Introduce 'worry time' and problem-solving if worrying is getting out of control.
- If you are feeling low and/or anxious a lot of the time, do visit your GP. There are many very good cancer charities and services that offer information, peer support, counselling and psychological support (see Resources).

Box 7.1

Although recovering well following breast cancer treatment, Jane realised that she still felt very anxious about the future, especially when she was tired or stressed. At these times she felt that she wouldn't be able to cope if anything else happened to her or to her family. Thinking about other challenges in her life, Jane remembered that she had felt very anxious before her first child was born, thinking that she would never manage to juggle being a nurse and a mother. She realised that despite her anxiety, she did have the resources to manage at the time, and she had actually adapted quite well. After deciding to take some time out from her career when her children were small, she had been able to resume her career once the children were a bit older. She had enjoyed taking this break and spending valuable time with her family.

Reviewing progress and maintaining changes

This is the last week of the self-help guide and an opportunity to review your progress overall as well as think about what was helpful (or not) for you. Everyone is different, so it is important to have a personal view about what is helpful for your menopausal symptoms and well-being. You can plan how you might continue with changes or goals during the next few weeks and months. Look back at the model of hot flushes on page 86. You will have used strategies over the last few weeks that link in directly to parts of the model.

For example:

- identifying and modifying precipitants of hot flushes;
- relaxation and breathing;
- stress management and lifestyle changes;

- problem-solving;
- pacing activities and exercise;
- hot flushes: thoughts and behaviour;
- managing flushes in social situations;
- night sweats and sleep: thoughts and behaviour; and
- others.

Now that you have completed the programme, look back to pages 33–34 where you initially wrote down your views about menopause. Have these changed at all since completing the programme? If so, make a note of how these beliefs may now be different in the space provided and consider whether this change is positive:

. . . .
. . . .
. . . .

Every now and then, I'll just look back and see where I've come from and where I'm at now.

You will be able to write down a simple plan of what you would like to do to maintain changes over the next few weeks and months using the sheet on page 158.

Maintaining changes

Think about what worked for you and what was less helpful. Use this information to create a 'maintenance plan'. Imagine how you will put your plan into action over the next week – which means when, where and how often you will carry out your plans. The goals of your action plan should be simple, specific and achievable.

What did I find helpful and why?

. . . .
. . . .
. . . .
. . . .
. . . .

To help you think about steps you can take for your maintenance plan, we have added some ideas taken from the women we have worked with, who completed the CBT programme.

Managing triggers

When I'd go into hot or busy places, I'd carry a fan with me . . . use a wet wipe in some cases . . . put some cold water on my wrists or possibly even on my face.

I can't not drink alcohol if I'm out, but I know if I do I'll be sweating all night. So I'm aware of what's causing them. If I choose to have a drink at nine o'clock at night, then I know full well that I'm going to be hot. So I'm controlling it.

Using paced breathing

I know that I have now got the tools to deal with it. . . . [W]hen I can feel a hot flush coming on, [I know] not to panic about it, just to use my breathing exercises, to use my relaxation.

Use that breath; it's free and it's natural, it's just there waiting. Half the time you can be panicking and then you tend to 'stiffen up' and stop breathing. That breath, it can help anybody in any situation.

If I'm somewhere where I can stop for a moment and just relax and breathe more evenly, then I will do it then. Quite often I can't. . . . [I]f I'm driving, for example, I can't. But I will relax and will turn on the air con and open the window.

Managing stress

I'm focusing on my exercise. I try to do that three or four times a week and things. For me, that is a great stress relief and I actually look forward to going to my classes and I realize just how much I do feel de-stressed afterwards.

I enjoyed writing down nice things that had happened at the end of every day. It was a nice experience. . . . I really enjoyed doing that.

I decided to do a lot more walking. I mean I've always walked to a certain degree, but I've maintained that. I make sure that I do it, maybe not as much as I'd like to, or like to have the time to, but I do try to maintain that.

Initially it was difficult because I'm very busy at work, always have got something to do at home . . . but now

I just get myself a book and sit down, even if it is only ten minutes, make a cup of tea, read a chapter of my book or something. It's just allowing yourself to do that. And it fits in. . . . [Y]ou can do it, it doesn't take long.

Managing hot flushes and night sweats

I'm still having them but I don't let them worry me really. I just think, 'Here you come . . . gone in a minute' which is a good thing. People have worse things.

When I get that feeling I think 'well, at least I'm not dying' or 'at least I know it's the hot flush'. Or actually, 'great, I'm awake: I can get to the gym early'. So I have really challenged negative thinking. And I think it worked.

I think 'God, will this go on forever?', but if it does . . . if I'm still having hot flushes in 10 years' time I know that I will be able to cope with that. . . . I've now got to the point where if it starts, I just relax and think, 'let it wash over you'. . . . And I just stop what I'm doing for a minute just to let it go and then it will go.

I've been in so many situations where I say, 'don't mind me, I'm having a hot flush'. . . . I don't feel embarrassed to tell someone that I'm having one. I've met so many other people who are actually having hot flushes and I say 'oh, you look too young to be having hot flushes', so you can share experiences. So it's made me more aware and open and things.

At work I'm telling my colleagues and friends about the menopause and encouraging them to talk about it more openly if they want to. . . . [I]t's important that we don't try to hide it because of embarrassment. We need to educate everyone – men and women.

Sleep and night sweats

I can be in control of my environment like, for example, I make sure that the heater gets turned off at a reasonable time, and our bed has got a very low tog duvet. . . . [I]f I was on the Tube on a hot day I would carry water to keep myself hydrated.

I definitely now don't drink caffeine near bedtime. Probably not after about six in the evening, unless I'm out having a meal in which case I might have a cup of coffee afterwards. And I do notice the difference. It's twofold in that I'm probably waking less because of the caffeine and I'm probably having fewer night sweats.

I used to watch the news and if something was on the news that upset me, it would play on my mind. So now I don't watch the news at night. If I want to know what's going on, I buy a paper every day. . . . I just try to relax about an hour before I go to bed rather than watching TV.

When you get tired and you know you're not going to get a good night's sleep, and it's in your head, 'oh, I'm going to have a really bad night', you get more irritated. So now I go to bed and I think, 'well, we'll see. It might be a good night or it might not'.

Maintenance plan

The plans you have set out need to be realistic and may vary according to what else is going on in your life. For example, if you are going through a particularly stressful time, it can be helpful not to put yourself under too much pressure to make major changes – it would be more helpful to focus on looking after yourself until things get easier. The first week of the self-help guide may give you ideas about ways to look after yourself during challenging times.

Potential barriers:

. . . .
. . . .
. . . .
. . . .
. . . .

What I can do to overcome them:

. . . .
. . . .
. . . .
. . . .
. . . .

Also think about future barriers to maintaining changes in advance. For example, increased workload or family problems may mean that your attention is focused elsewhere for a time, and it is more difficult to keep up with your planned changes. Look back to page 93 and remind yourself of what your different signs of stress are. Spotting these early on can help you to feel a little bit more in control, as you can put in place coping strategies before everything gets on top of you.

Choose one or more of the helpful skills or activities that you have learned during the four weeks and write them down in the table provided. Refer to this plan to keep you on track.

Maintenance Plan 1 (This might include anything to do with habits, activities, behaviour changes and ways of thinking.)
What?
When?
Where?
Maintenance Plan 2
What?
When?
Where?

Box 7.2

Jane's potential barriers to maintaining changes were: (i) an increase in her workload or increased work stress and (ii) not getting enough time for herself.

Jane chose the following maintenance strategies to put into action:

1 What? Keep calm and breathe for a few minutes or until

I start to calm down.

When? When I notice myself getting stressed.

Where? Wherever I am.

2 What? Be aware of tendency to catastrophize, leading to anxiety, and use the thought strategies to remain calm.

When? When my mood becomes anxious or low.

Where? Wherever I am or later at home when I can reflect and work through the questions if needs be.

3 What? Only do what is manageable at these times. This means saying no to some tasks and prioritizing time for myself (an hour a day) and time to relax (20 mins a day).

When? When I notice increased workload or work stress and when I am not getting enough time for myself.

Where? At work and at home, in the evening.

Week 4 Homework
- Keep practising the relaxation and breathing and use it to help deal with stress, hot flushes and sleep and night sweats.
- Put your maintenance plan into action.
- Please fill in the Hot Flush Rating Scale and diary for Week 4.

RELAX → SLOW BREATHING → CALMING THOUGHTS

GOOD LUCK!

Table 7.1 Hot flush diary, Week 4 Date:

	Monday	Tuesday	Wednesday	Thursday	Friday	Saturday	Sunday
1–6 a.m.							
6–9 a.m.							
9–12 a.m.							
12–2 p.m.							
2–4 p.m.							
4–6 p.m.							
6–8 p.m.							
8–10 p.m.							
10–12 p.m.							

Printable copies of the diaries in this book are available to download; visit the 'eResources' site: www.routledge.com/9780367853037

Hot flush rating scale

When you have finished the self-help guide (usually four to six weeks after you began), you can rate your hot flushes so that you can see whether they have changed.

1 How often have you had hot flushes in the past week?
Please estimate: . . . . times each day, or . . . . times each week

2 If you have night sweats, how often have they woken you up in the past week?
Please estimate: . . . . times each day, or . . . . times each week

Please circle a number on each scale to indicate how your flushes/sweats have been during the past week:

3 To what extent do you regard your flushes/sweats as a problem?
No problem at all   Very much a problem

1 2 3 4 5 6 7 8 9 10

4 How distressed do you feel about your hot flushes?
Not distressed at all   Very distressed indeed

1 2 3 4 5 6 7 8 9 10

5 How much do your hot flushes interfere with your daily routine?
Not at all   Very much indeed

1 2 3 4 5 6 7 8 9 10

Add up the numbers of hot flushes and night sweats in the past week which gives your
Hot flush frequency total score = ...
and add up the scores on numbers 3, 4 and 5 and divide by

3. This will give you your

Problem-rating score = ...

In our research trials, the problem rating scores were the main measures that we aimed to change because it is the hot flush problem rating that is commonly associated with quality of life: it is the extent to which hot flushes and night sweats are problematic that determines whether women seek help or not. On average, women came into the studies having 70 hot flushes and night sweats each week, and these reduced typically to around 50 after CBT and to approximately 45 at the follow-up assessment four to six months later. In terms of the problem rating scores, these were on average 6 to 7 out of 10 before the CBT; afterwards, they were reduced to around 3 out of 10, reflecting flushes that had become much less bothersome (Ayers *et al*. 2012; Mann *et al*. 2012). Again, the improvements were maintained four to six months later. You can compare these scores with your own scores at the beginning and at the end of the self-help guide. We hope that you gained some benefits too.

These are, of course, averages, and some women benefited more than others. In more recent analyses of the trials, it seems that if you were coping very well before the CBT, or if you had a very healthy lifestyle with plenty of exercise and low levels of stress, you might have less to work on and might not notice such large improvements. The extent of benefit will also be related to how much time and commitment that you have been able to put into the self-help exercises. However, you can always go back to it as needed.

We interviewed women after the end of the studies to find out what they thought about the self-help CBT and what changes they experienced (Balabanovic et al. 2012, 2013).

We found that the women who used the self-help CBT did comment on the need for motivation and the self-directed learning, and those who were more motivated found it easiest to deal with. Nevertheless, it was as effective in reducing the impact of hot flushes and night sweats as group CBT where women met for four weekly two-hour sessions.

I'm such a disciplined person. . . . It suited me exactly and I knew it would. I thought 'this is going to help me and I need to do this on my own'. . . . Every evening I sat down and I did my exercises.

In contrast, women who were less disciplined or who were more time-constrained (e.g. working full time) sometimes struggled to work through the entire booklet.

Well, the times that I did it [relaxation], I had to stay up late at night. Sometimes I fell asleep. . . . I didn't quite finish doing them for that reason; you know, finding the time.

Some also appreciated having their booklet nearby for future reference.

I keep it by my bedside. . . . [E]very now and then I'll just look back and see where I've come from and where I'm at now.

Although many women reported reduced frequency of hot flushes and night sweats, the majority described the main change as reduced symptom severity or impact.

I'm not sure whether they've got worse or better, or whether I just don't think about them as often. Sometimes I think 'oh, maybe I've had hot flushes' and I don't even realize I've had one.

Although you can't do much about the frequency of them, you can actually do something about the severity of them. You can either get yourself into a tizzy over it or you can let it go over you.

Most women described several main benefits of working through the process, such as learning strategies to cope with hot flushes and night sweats, increased knowledge and understanding of menopause and hot flushes, feeling more relaxed generally and regaining a sense of control.

I would say that it's been excellent for me. I initially thought that I could do absolutely nothing to help myself with menopausal symptoms. . . . [G]oing through the book and realizing that I could control things has been excellent for me. . . . I hardly have any hot flushes now.

One woman was planning her return to work following treatment for breast cancer when she started having CBT for her flushes:

I was thinking 'how on earth can I start back at work without feeling totally useless?' because of all these symptoms. But now I can control them better and also feel more confident in general.

Many of the women felt that their ability to cope with hot flushes had improved due to their being better informed about the flushes as well as having developed a more accepting stance towards the symptoms (allowing the flush to run its course, for example, or 'letting it go').

The hot sweats vary during the day, they come and go, [but] understanding them helps. . . . [I]t's coping with them that has become easier.

For some reason, maybe because I've come to accept them, they seem to be less frequent and less severe, you know; they seem to be quite mild.

Resources

Menopause

International Menopause Society
The aims of the IMS are to promote knowledge, study and research on all aspects of ageing in men and women; to organize, prepare, hold and participate in international meetings and congresses on menopause; and to encourage the interchange of research plans and experience between individual members.

www.imsociety.org
IMS Executive Director
PO Box 98
Camborne
Cornwall, UK TR14 4BQ
Tel: +44 (0)1209 711 054
Email: leetomkinsims@btinternet.com

British Menopause Society
The British Menopause Society (BMS) is a registered charity and multidisciplinary society for women seeking information and advice as well as nurses and doctors and other health professional. Although primarily a professional organisation, the BMS website includes information aimed at the general public, including a number of fact sheets on various aspects of the menopause.

www.thebms.org.uk
British Menopause Society
4–6 Eton Place
Marlow
Buckinghamshire, UK SL7 2QA
Tel: +44 (0) 1628 890199
Fax: +44 (0) 1628 474042

North American Menopause Society

The North American Menopause Society (NAMS) is a leading non-profit organisation dedicated to promoting the health and quality of life of women during midlife and beyond through an understanding of menopause and healthy ageing. Its multidisciplinary membership includes clinical and basic science experts from medicine, nursing, sociology, psychology, nutrition, anthropology, epidemiology, pharmacy and education and enables NAMS to provide balanced information. Includes sections for health professionals as well as women experiencing menopause. It publishes the journal *Menopause Management*.

www.menopause.org
5900 Landerbrook Drive
Suite 390
Mayfield Heights, OH 44124, USA
Tel: +1 440 442 7550
Email: info@menopause.org

Menopause Exchange (newsletter and website)

The Menopause Exchange gives independent advice and is not sponsored by commercial organisations. It provides information on a range of topics, including menopausal symptoms, osteoporosis, self-help measures, HRT, alternatives to HRT and products. Its 'Ask the Experts' panel includes many of the UK's top healthcare professionals working in the field of the menopause. The site features a blog and online articles.

www.menopause-exchange.co.uk
The Menopause Exchange
PO Box 205
Bushey, Herts, UK WD23 1ZS
Tel: +44 (0) 20 8420 7245
Fax: +44 (0) 20 8954 2783
Email: info@menopause-exchange.co.uk

Menopause Support

A not-for-profit enterprise helping women to share remedies, advice and information based on their own experience. Its website includes a blog and suggestions for dietary change. It also offers workshops and one-to-one telephone advice as well as Facebook and Twitter accounts.

www.menopausesupport.org.uk
Tel: +44 (0) 1392 876122
Email: info@menopausesupport.org.uk

Menopause Matters

An independent website providing up-to-date, accurate information about the menopause, menopausal symptoms and treatment options. It offers information on what happens leading up to, during and after the menopause; what the consequences can be; what you can do to help; and what treatments are available. You can keep in touch via its Facebook and Twitter accounts.

www.menopausematters.co.uk

The Daisy Network

The Daisy Network Premature Menopause Support Group is a registered UK charity for women who have experienced a premature menopause. It is a not-for-profit organisation. The website provides information about premature menopause and the issues around it.

www.daisynetwork.org.uk
The Daisy Network
PO Box 183
Rossendale, Lancashire, UK BB4 6WZ

Fertility Friends

Fertility Friends is a web-based information and support community. Its message boards allow you to ask a nurse and other relevant professionals questions or to chat with other people affected by infertility.

General women's health and well-being

Women's Health Concern

Women's Health Concern is the UK's leading charity providing help and advice to women on a wide variety of health, well-being and lifestyle concerns, to enable them to work in partnership with their own medical practitioners. Information is offered by telephone, email, in print, online and through conferences, seminars and symposia.

www.womens-health-concern.org
4–6 Eton Place
Marlow, Bucks, UK SL7 2QA
Tel (office): +44 (0) 1628 478 473
Advice line: +44 (0) 845 123231

Women's Health London
Telephone helpline offering assistance on various aspects of women's health.

www.womenshealthlondon.org.uk.
52 Featherstone Street
London EC1Y 8RT
Helpline: +44 (0) 845 125 5254
Tel. +44 (0) 20 7251 6333
Fax: +44 (0) 20 7250 4152
Email: health@womenshealthlondon.org.uk

Women's Health
Online site offering information and forums around all aspects of women's health including many aspects of menopause.

www.womens-health.co.uk

NHS Live Well
An NHS website offering health and well-being advice including real stories and online assessment tools for all ages, but with specific sections for women aged 40 to 60 and 60+, including many aspects of menopause as well as keeping healthy.

www.nhs.uk/LiveWell/Women4060/Pages/Women4060home.aspx

Breast Cancer Care
This charity offers information and offer emotional and practical support to people.

www.breastcancercare.org.uk/
Helpline: +44 (0) 808 800 6000
Email: info@breastcancercare.org.uk

Cancer Research UK
Its website provides information about all types of cancer, spotting early symptoms, and the emotional consequences of

a cancer diagnosis. Also provided are an e-newsletter, Twitter posts, blogs and podcasts. The charity funds research into cancer and provides telephone helpline support.

www.cancerresearchuk.org
Angel Building
407 St John Street
London EC1V 4AD
Tel: (Supporter Services): +44 (0)300 123 1022
Tel: (Switchboard): +44 (0)20 7242 0200

Macmillan Cancer Support
Provides practical, medical and financial support and campaigns for better cancer care via its website and local groups. It also offers an online community for people diagnosed with cancer and carers.

www.macmillan.org.uk
89 Albert Embankment
London SE1 7UQ
Helpline: +44 (0)808 808 00 00

National osteoporosis society
Offers information about osteoporosis through a range of booklets, magazines, telephone helpline and regional support groups.

www.nos.org.uk
Camerton
Bath BA2 0PJ
Tel: +44 (0)1761 471771 or +44 (0) 845 130 3076
Email: info@nos.org.uk

Menopause in the workplace
Guidelines on Menopause in the workplace:
Trades Union Congress, 2013
www.tuc.org.uk/resource/supporting-working-women-through-menopause
Chartered Institute of Personnel and Development (CIPD), 2019 The Menopause at Work: a practical guide for people managers. www.cipd.co.uk
Faculty of Occupational Medicine – www.fom.ac.uk/health-at-work-2/information-for-employers/dealing-with-health-problems-in-the-workplace/advice-on-the-menopause

Online support groups

Henpicked, Menopause in the Workplace – https://menopau seintheworkplace.co.uk

Menopause Café – 'gather to eat cake, drink tea and discuss menopause' – www.menopausecafe.net

Talking Menopause – www.talkingmenopause.co.uk

Menopause Support – https://menopausesupport.co.uk/

Twitter sites

Behind the woman Midlife health and well-being @behind the woman

aims to reduce the negative images of menopausal women.

Working with the menopause @menopausecbt

provides workplace education for employees and managers and CBT for women.

Mental health and self-help tools

www.iapt.nhs.uk

For details of Increasing Access to Psychological Therapy (IAPT) services in your area, please go to www.nhs.uk/service-search/counselling-nhs-(iapt)-services/locationsearch/396 and enter your town/postcode. You can also contact your GP for a referral.

www.moodjuice.scot.nhs.uk/

Moodjuice is an internet site developed by Choose Life Falkirk and the Adult Clinical Psychology Service, NHS Forth Valley. The site is designed to offer information and advice to those experiencing troublesome thoughts, feelings and actions. From the site you are able to print off various self-help guides covering conditions such as depression, anxiety, stress, panic and sleep problems.

www.ntw.nhs.uk/pic/selfhelp

Northumberland, Tyne and Wear NHS Foundation Trust is one of the largest mental health and disability Trusts in England and provides downloadable CBT-based self-help guides for conditions including anxiety, panic, anger, obsessions and compulsions and bereavement.

www.rcpsych.ac.uk/expertadvice.aspx

Readable, user-friendly and accurate information about mental health problems, including signposting to relevant services.

www.mind.org.uk/

Mind publishes information on many topics relating to mental health, grouped into seven broad categories: diagnoses and conditions, treatments, mental health statistics, support and social care, communities and social groups, society and environment.

PO Box 277
Manchester M60 3XN
Tel: +44 (0)300 123 3393
Email: info@mind.org.uk

Psychotherapy

BRITISH PSYCHOLOGICAL SOCIETY
The British Psychological Society is the representative body for psychology and psychologists in the UK. It is responsible for the development, promotion and application of psychology.

www.bps.org.uk/psychology-public/find-psychologist/
find-psychologist
www.counselling.co.uk
1 Regent Place
Rugby, Warks, UK CV21 2PJ
Tel: +44 (0) 870 443 5252
Fax: +44 (0)870 443 5160
Email: bac@bac.co.uk

British association for behavioural and cognitive psychotherapy
A lead organisation for CBT in the UK and Ireland. Its website includes a register of accredited CBT therapists.

www.babcp.com
Imperial House
Hornby Street
Bury, Lancashire, UK BL9 5BN
Tel: +44 (0) 161 705 4304

The Samaritans
Helpline offering emotional support for anyone in a crisis

www.samaritans.org.uk
10 The Grove
Slough, UK SL1 1QP
Helpline: +44 (0)845 790 9090
Fax: +44 (0)1753 819 004
Email: jo@samaritans.org.uk

Turn2me

An online mental health community offering peer and professional support for people suffering from anxiety and depression, including online CBT tools, a blog, information articles, and podcasts.

www.turn2me.org
Turn2MeUK
1 Pendlebury
Hamworth
Bracknell, Berks, UK RG12 7RB

Anxiety

NO PANIC
   The National Organisation for Phobias, Anxiety, Neurosis, Information and Care. Its website has a range of downloadable information booklets.

www.nopanic.org.uk
Unit 3
Prospect House
Halesfield 22
Telford, Shrops TF7 4QX
Tel: +44 (0)1952 680460
Email: ceo@nopanic.org.uk

Depression

The depression alliance

The website contains information about the symptoms of depression, treatments for depression, as well as research, publications, campaigns, and local self-help groups.

www.depressionalliance.org/
20 Great Dover Street
London SE1 4LX
Email: information@depressionalliance.org

Miscellaneous support

Relate
Relationship counselling.

> www.relate.org.uk
> Herbert Gray College
> Little Church Street
> Rugby CV21 3AP
> Tel: +44 (0)1788 573241
> Fax: +44 (0) 1788 535007

Carers UK
Information and advice on all aspects of caring.

> www.carersuk.demon.co.uk
> 20–25 Glasshouse Yard
> London EC1A 4JT
> Carers' line: 0808 808 7777
> Tel: +44 (0) 20 7490 8818
> Fax: +44 (0) 20 7490 8824
> Email: info@ukcarers.org

Careline
Telephone counselling on any issue.

> Cardinal Heenan Centre
> 326 High Road
> Ilford, Essex IG1 1QP
> Helpline: +44 (0) 20 8514 1177
> Office tel: +44 (0) 8514 5444
> Fax: +44 (0) 20 8478 7943
> Email: careline@totalise.co.uk

Cruse bereavement care
Provides support services for people who have been bereaved.

> www.crusebereavementcare.org.uk
> 126 Sheen Road
> Richmond, Surrey TW9 1UR
> Helpline: 0870 167 1677
> Office tel: +44 (0) 20 8939 9530
> Fax: +44 (0) 20 8939 9530
> Email: info@crusebereavementcare.org.uk

Divorce Support Group (DSG)

A professionally run organisation providing local support groups and individual support to help you cope with the emotional and psychological impact of your divorce or separation.

www.divorcesupportgroup.co.uk
Tel: +44 (0) 844 800 90 98
Email: mail@divorcesupportgroup.co.uk

The Athena Network

A networking site for women, which aims to help members link up across a range of industry sectors.

theathenanetwork.co.uk
30 Northfield Gardens
Watford, Herts, UK WD24 7RE
Email: enquiries@theathenanetwork.co.uk.

References

Abernethy, K. (2018) *Menopause: the one-stop guide*. London: Profile Books.

Agency for Health Research and Quality (AHRQ). (2012) *Medicine for Treating Depression: A Review of the Research for Adults*. AHRQ Pub No. 12-EHC012-A. Department of Health and Human Services.

American Society of Clinical Oncology. (2019) Accessed at www.cancer.net/coping-with-cancer/physical-emotional-and-social-effects-cancer/managing-physical-side-effects/weight-gain.

Anderson, L., Lewis, G., Araya, R., Elgie, R., Harrison, G., Proudfoot, J. *et al*. (2005) Self-help books for depression: How can practitioners and patients make the right choice? *The British Journal of General Practice*, 55(514): 387.

Andrikoula, M. and Prevelic, G. (2009) Menopausal hot flushes revisited. *Climacteric*, 12: 3–15.

Archer, D.F., Sturdee, D.W., Baber, R., de Villiers, T.J., Pines, A., Freedman, R.R. *et al*. (2011) Menopausal hot flushes and night sweats: Where are we now? *Climacteric*, 14(5): 515–528.

Atema, V., van Leeuwen, M., Kieffer, J.M., Oldenburg, H.S.A., van Beurden, M., Gerritsma, M.A. *et al*. (2019) Efficacy of internet-based cognitive behavioral therapy for treatment-induced menopausal symptoms in breast cancer survivors: Results of a randomized controlled trial. *Journal of Clinical Oncology*, 37. https://doi.org/10.1200/JCO.18.00655.

A-tjak, J.G., Davis, M.L., Morina, N., Powers, M.B., Smits, J.A. and Emmelkamp, P.M. (2015) A meta-analysis of the efficacy of acceptance and commitment therapy for clinically relevant mental and physical health problems. *Psychotherapy and Psychosomatics*, 84(1): 30–36.

Avis, N.E., Crawford, S.L., Greendale, G., Bromberger, J.T., Everson-Rose, S.A., Gold, E.B. *et al*. (2015) Duration of menopausal vasomotor symptoms over the menopause transition. *Journal of the American Medical Association Internal Medicine*, 175(4): 531–539.

Avis, N.E., Crawford, S.L. and McKinley, S.M. (1997) Psycho-social behavioural and health factors related to menopause symptomatology. *Women's Health*, 3(2): 103–120.

Avis, N.E. and McKinlay, S.M. (1991) A longitudinal analysis of women's attitudes toward the menopause: Results from the Massachusetts women's health study. *Maturitas*, 13: 65–79.

Avis, N.E., Ory, M., Matthews, K.M., Schocken, M., Bromberger, J. and Colvin, A. (2003) Health-related quality of life in a multiethnic sample of middle-aged women: Study of Women's health across the nation (SWAN). *Medical Care*, 41(11): 1262–1276.

Avis, N.E., Stellato, R., Crawford, J., Bromberger, J., Ganz, P., Cain, V. *et al.* (2001) Is there a menopausal syndrome? Menopausal status and symptoms across racial/ethnic groups. *Social Science and Medicine*, 52: 345–356.

Avis, N.E., Stellato, R., Crawford, S.L., Johannes, C.B. and Longcope, C. (2000) Is there an association between menopause status and sexual functioning? *Menopause*, 7(5): 297–309.

Avis, N.E., Zhao, X., Johannes, C., Ory, M., Brockwell, S. and Greendale, G. (2005) Correlates of sexual function among multi-ethnic middle-aged women: Results from the study of women's health across the nation (SWAN). *Menopause*, 12(4): 385–398.

Ayers, B., Forshaw, M. and Hunter, M.S. (2010) The impact of attitudes towards the menopause on women's symptom experience: A systematic review. *Maturitas*, 65: 28–36.

Ayers, B. and Hunter, M.S. (2012) Health-related quality of life of women with menopausal hot flushes and night sweats. *Climacteric*, 15: 1–5.

Ayers, B., Smith, M., Hellier, J., Mann, E. and Hunter, M.S. (2012) Effectiveness of group and self-help cognitive behaviour therapy to reduce problematic menopausal hot flushes and night sweats (MENOS 2): A randomized controlled trial. *Menopause: Journal of the North American Menopause Society*, 19: 749–759.

Balabanovic, J., Ayers, B. and Hunter, M.S. (2012) Cognitive behaviour therapy for menopausal hot flushes and night sweats: A qualitative analysis of women's experiences of group and self-help CBT. *Behavioural and Cognitive Psychotherapy*, 1(1): 1–17.

Balabanovic, J., Ayers, B. and Hunter, M.S. (2013) An exploration of women's experiences of group cognitive behaviour therapy to treat breast cancer treatment-related hot flushes and night sweats: An interpretative phenomenological analysis. *Maturitas*, 72(3): 236–242.

Bandura, A. (1995) *Self-efficacy in changing societies*. New York: Cambridge University Press.

Beck, A.T. (1976) *Cognitive therapy and the emotional disorders.* Oxford: International Universities Press.

Beck, A.T., Rush, A.J., Shaw, B.F. and Emery, G. (1979) *Cognitive therapy of depression.* New York: Guilford Press.

Befus, D., Coeytaux, R.R., Goldstein, K.M., McDuffie, J.R., Shepherd-Banigan, M., Goode, A.P. *et al.* (2018) Management of menopause symptoms with acupuncture: An umbrella systematic review and meta-analysis. *Journal of Alternative and Complementary Medicine*, 24(4): 314–323.

Bellott, E., Rouse, N. and Hunter, M.S. (2018) Reclaim the menopause: A pilot study of an evidence-based menopause course for symptom management in resilience building. *Post Reproductive Health*, 24(2): 79–81.

Beral, V. (2003) Breast cancer and hormone replacement therapy in the million women study. *Lancet*, 362: 419–427.

Berin, E., Hammar, M., Lindblom, H., Lindh-Åstrand, L., Rubér, M. and Holm, A.C.S. (2019) Resistance training for hot flushes in postmenopausal women: A randomised controlled trial. *Maturitas*, 126: 55–60.

Beyene, Y.C. (1986) Cultural significance and physiological manifestations of the menopause: A biocultural analysis. *Culture, Medicine and Psychiatry*, 10: 47–71.

Blenkiron, P. (2005) Stories and analogies in cognitive behaviour therapy: A clinical review. *Behavioural and Cognitive Psychotherapy*, 33(1): 45–59.

Bonnet, M.J. (1990) The perception of sleep onset in insomniacs and normal sleepers. In Bootzin, R.R., Kihlstrom, J.F. and Schacter, D.L. (Eds.) *Sleep and Cognition.* Washington, DC: American Psychological Association, pp. 148–158, ix, 211.

Borkovec, T.D. (1982) Insomnia. *Journal of Consulting and Clinical Psychology*, 50(6): 880–895.

Borrelli, F. and Ernst, E. (2010) Alternative and complementary therapies for the menopause. *Maturitas*, 66(4): 333–343.

Brown, L., Brown, V., Judd, F. and Bryant, C. (2017) It's not as bad as you think: Menopausal representations are more positive in postmenopausal women. *Journal of Psychosomatic Obstetrics & Gynecology*, 39(4): 281–288.

Brown, L., Bryant, C. and Judd, F.K. (2015) Positive well-being during the menopausal transition: A systematic review. *Climacteric*, 18(4): 456–469.

Burger, H.G. (2006) Physiology and endocrinology of the menopause. *Medicine*, 34(1): 27–30.

Busch, H., Barth-Olofsson, A.S., Rosenhagen, S. and Collins, A. (2003) Menopausal transition and psychological development. *Menopause*, 10(2): 179–187.

Campbell, K.E., Dennerstein, L., Finch, S. and Szoeke, C.E. (2017) Impact of menopausal status on negative mood and depressive symptoms in a longitudinal sample spanning 20 years. *Menopause*, 24(5): 490–496.

Carpenter, J., Johnson, D., Wagner, L. and Andrykowski, M. (2002) Hot flashes and related outcomes in breast cancer survivors and matched comparison women. *Oncology Nursing Forum*, 29(3): 16–25.

Chalder, T. (1995) *Coping with chronic fatigue*. London: Sheldon Press.

Chambers, D., Bagnall, A.M., Hempel, S. and Forbes, C. (2006) Interventions for the treatment, management and rehabilitation of patients with chronic fatigue syndrome/myalgic encephalomyelitis: An updated systematic review. *Journal of the Royal Society of Medicine*, 99(10): 506–520.

Chilcot, J., Norton, S. and Hunter, M.S. (2014) Cognitive behaviour therapy for menopausal symptoms following breast cancer treatment: Who benefits and how does it work? *Maturitas*, 78(1): 56–61.

Clark, D.M. (1986) A cognitive approach to panic. *Behaviour Research and Therapy*, 24(4): 461–470.

Clark, D.M. and Wells, A. (1995) A cognitive model of social phobia. In Heimberg, R.G., Liebowitz, M.R., Hope, D.A. and Schneier, F.R. (Eds.) *Social Phobia: Diagnosis, Assessment, and Treatment*. New York: Guilford Press, pp. 69–93, xii.

Col, N.F., Guthrie, J.R., Politi, M. and Dennerstein, L. (2009) Duration of vasomotor symptoms in middle aged women: A longitudinal study. *Menopause*, 16: 453–457.

Davis, S.R., Castelo-Branco, C., Chedraui, P., Lumsden, M.A., Nappi, R.E., Shah, D. *et al.* (2012) Understanding weight gain at menopause. *Climacteric*, 15: 419–429.

Dennerstein, L., Guthrie, J.R., Clark, M., Lehert, P. and Henderson, V.W. (2004) A population-based study of depressed mood in middle-aged, Australian-born women. *Menopause*, 11(5): 563–568.

Dennerstein, L., Lehert, P. and Burger, H. (2005) The relative effects of hormones and relationship factors on sexual function of women through the natural menopausal transition. *Fertility and Sterility*, 84(10): 174–180.

Department of Health. (2008) *IAPT Implementation Plan: National Guidelines for Regional Delivery*. Available at www.iapt.nhs.uk.

Deutsch, H. (1945) *The psychology of women*. Oxford: Grune and Stratton.

Devlin, R. (2019) *Men let's talk menopause: what's going on and what you can do about it*. Practical Inspiration Publishing.

Duijts, S.F.A., van Beurden, M., Oldenburg, H.S.A., Hunter, M.S., Kieffer, J.M., Stuiver, M.M. *et al.* (2012) Efficacy of cognitive behavioral therapy and physical exercise in alleviating treatment-induced menopausal symptoms in patients with breast cancer: Results of a randomized, controlled, multicenter trial. *Journal of Clinical Oncology*, 30(33): 4124–4133.

Edwards, D. and Panay, N. (2016) Treating vulvovaginal atrophy/genitourinary syndrome of menopause: How important is vaginal lubricant and moisturizer composition? *Climacteric*, 19(2): 151–161.

Eichling, P.S., Freedman, R., Polo-Kantola, P. and Shaver, J. (2005) Menopause and sleep. *Menopause Management*, 14: 25–29.

Ellis, M. (2007) Current and future choices in endocrine therapy. *Breast Cancer Research*, 9(2): S15.

Espie, C.A. (2010) *Overcoming insomnia and sleep problems*. London: Constable and Robinson.

Eziefula, C., Grunfeld, E.A. and Hunter, M.S. (2013) 'You know I've joined your club . . . I'm the hot flush boy': A qualitative exploration of hot flushes in men undergoing androgen deprivation therapy for prostate cancer. *Psychooncology*, 22(12): 2823–2830.

Falleti, M.G., Sanfilippo, A., Maruff, P., Weih, L. and Phillips, K.A. (2005) The nature and severity of cognitive impairment associated with adjuvant chemotherapy in women with breast cancer: A meta-analysis of the current literature. *Brain and Cognition*, 59(1): 60–70.

Fenlon, D.R., Corner, J.L. and Haviland, J. (2009) Menopausal hot flushes after breast cancer. *European Journal of Cancer Care*, 18: 140–148.

Fenlon, D.R. and Rogers, A.E. (2007) The experience of hot flushes after breast cancer. *Cancer Nursing*, 30(4): 19–26.

Fennell, M. (2016) *Overcoming low self-esteem: a self-help guide using cognitive behavioural techniques*. London: Robinson.

Ferguson, R.J., Ahles, T.A., Saykin, A.J., McDonald, B.C., Furstenberg, C.T., Cole, B.F. and Mott, L.A. (2007) Cognitive-behavioral management of chemotherapy-related cognitive change. *Psycho-Oncology*, 16(8): 772–777.

Ferrie, J.E., Shipley, M.J., Cappuccio, F.P., Brunner, E., Miller, M.A., Kumari, M. *et al.* (2007) A prospective study of change in sleep duration: Associations with mortality in the Whitehall II cohort. *Sleep*, 30(12): 1659.

Finn, C.A. (2002) Why do women have menopause? *Journal of the British Menopause Society*, 8(1): 10–14.

Flint, M. (1975) The menopause: Reward or punishment? *Psychosomatics*, 16: 161–163.

Ford, N., Slade, P. and Butler, G. (2005) An absence of evidence linking perceived memory problems to the menopause. *British Journal of General Practice*, 54: 434–438.

Franco, O.H., Chowdhury, R., Troup, J., Voortman, T., Kunutsor, S. *et al*. (2016) Use of plant-based therapies and menopausal symptoms: A systematic review and meta-analysis. *Journal of the American Medical Association*, 315: 2554–2563.

Freedman, R.R. (2005) Pathophysiology and treatment of menopausal hot flashes. *Seminars in Reproductive Medicine*, 23: 117–125.

Freedman, R.R. and Krell, W. (1999) Reduced thermoregulatory null zone in postmenopausal women with hot flashes. *American Journal of Obstetrics and Gynecology*, 181: 66–70.

Freeman, E.W., Sammel, M.D., Lin, H., Gracia, C.R., Kapoor, S. and Ferdousi, T. (2005) The role of anxiety and hormonal changes in menopausal hot flashes. *Menopause*, 12(3): 258–266.

Freeman, E.W., Sammel, M.D., Lin, H., Liu, Z. and Gracia, C.R. (2011) Duration of menopausal hot flushes and associated risk factors. *Obstetrics Gynecology*, 117(5): 1095–1104.

Freeman, E.W. and Sherif, K. (2007) Prevalence of hot flushes and night sweats around the world: A systematic review. *Climacteric*, 10: 197–214.

Gannon, L., Hansel, S. and Goodwin, J. (1987) Correlates of menopausal hot flashes. *Journal of Behavioral Medicine*, 10: 277–285.

Gatchel, R.J. and Rollings, K.H. (2008) Evidence-informed management of chronic low back pain with cognitive behavioral therapy. *The Spine Journal*, 8(1): 40–44.

Gilbert, P. (2009) *The compassionate mind*. London: Constable and Robinson.

Gold, E.B., Colvin, A., Avis, N., Bromberger, J., Greendale, G.A., Powell, L. *et al*. (2006) Longitudinal analysis of the association between vasomotor symptoms and race/ethnicity across the menopausal transition: Study of women's health across the nation (SWAN). *American Journal of Public Health*, 96: 1226–1235.

Green, S.M., Donegan, E., Frey, B.N., Key, B.L., Fredorkow, D., Streiner, D.L.L. *et al*. (2019) Cognitive behavior therapy for menopausal symptoms (CBT-Meno): A randomized controlled trial. *Menopause*, 26(9): 972–980.

Griffiths, A. and Hunter, M.S. (2015) Psychosocial factors and menopause: The impact of menopause on personal and working life. In Davies, S.C. (Ed.) *Annual Report of the Chief Medical Officer 2014, the Health of 51%*. London: Department of Health.

Gupta, P., Sturdee, D.W. and Hunter, M.S. (2006a) Mid-aged health in women from the Indian subcontinent (MAHWIS): General health and the experience of the menopause in women. *Climacteric*, 9(1): 13–22.

Gupta, P., Sturdee, D.W., Palin, S., Majumder, K., Fear, R., Marshall, T. *et al.* (2006b) Menopausal symptoms in women treated for breast cancer: The prevalence and severity of symptoms and their perceived effects on quality of life. *Climacteric*, 9(1): 49–58.

Hanisch, L.J., Hantsoo, L., Freeman, E.W., Sullivan, G.M. and Coyne, J.C. (2008) Hot flashes and panic attacks: A comparison of symptomatology, neurobiology, treatment, and a role for cognition. *Psychological Bulletin*, 134(2): 247–269.

Hardy, C., Griffiths, A. and Hunter, M.S. (2017) What do working menopausal women want? A qualitative investigation into women's perspectives on employer and line manager support. *Maturitas*, 101: 37–41.

Hardy, C., Griffiths, A. and Hunter, M.S. (2019) Development and evaluation of online menopause awareness training for line managers in UK organizations. *Maturitas*, 120: 83–89.

Hardy, C., Griffiths, A., Norton, S. and Hunter, M.S. (2018a) Self-help cognitive behavior therapy for working women with problematic hot flushes and night sweats (MENOS@Work): A multicenter randomized controlled trial. *Menopause*, 25(5): 508–519.

Hardy, C., Thorne, E., Griffiths, A. and Hunter, M.S. (2018b) Work outcomes in midlife women: The impact of menopause, work stress and working environment. *Women's Midlife Health*, 4: 3–8.

Harkness, E., Macdonald, W., Valderas, J., Coventry, P., Gask, L. and Bower, P. (2010) Identifying psychosocial interventions that improve both physical and mental health in patients with diabetes: A systematic review and meta-analysis. *Diabetes Care*, 33(4): 926–930.

Harlow, S.D., Gass, M., Hall, J.E., Lobo, R., Maki, P., Rebar, R.W. *et al.* (2012) Executive summary of the stages of reproductive aging workshop +10: Addressing the unfinished agenda of staging reproductive aging. *Menopause*, 19(4): 105–114.

Harvey, A.G. (2002) A cognitive model of insomnia. *Behaviour Research and Therapy*, 40(8): 869–893.

Hayes, S.C., Follette, V.M. and Lineham, M.M. (2004) *Mindfulness and acceptance: expanding the cognitive behavioural tradition*. New York: Guilford Press.

Henderson, V.W. (2009) Menopause, cognitive aging and dementia: Practice implications. *Menopause International*, 15: 41–44.

Hickey, M., Szabo, R.A. and Hunter, M.S. (2017) Non-hormonal treatments for menopausal symptoms. *British Medical Journal*, 359: J5101.

Hill, K. (1996) The demography of menopause. *Maturitas*, 23: 113–127.

Høifødt, R.S., Strøm, C., Kolstrup, N., Eisemann, M. and Waterloo, K. (2011) Effectiveness of cognitive behavioural therapy in primary health care: A review. *Family Practice*, 28(5): 489–504.

Hofmann, S.G., Sawyer, A.T. and Fang, A. (2010) The empirical status of the 'new wave' of CBT. *The Psychiatric Clinics of North America*, 33(3): 701.

Hofmann, S.G. and Smits, J.A. (2008) Cognitive-behavioral therapy for adult anxiety disorders: A meta-analysis of randomized placebo-controlled trials. *The Journal of Clinical Psychiatry*, 69(4): 621.

Hunter, M.S. (2003) Cognitive behavioural interventions for premenstrual and menopausal problems. *Journal of Reproductive and Infant Psychology*, 21: 183–194.

Hunter, M.S., Ayers, B. and Smith, M. (2011) The hot flush behaviour scale: A measure of behavioural reactions to menopausal hot flushes and night sweats. *Menopause*, 18(11): 178–183.

Hunter, M.S., Coventry, S., Mendes, N. and Grunfeld, E.A. (2009a) Evaluation of a group cognitive behavioural intervention for women suffering from menopausal symptoms following breast cancer treatment. *Psycho-Oncology*, 18: 560–563.

Hunter, M.S., Coventry, S., Mendes, N. and Grunfeld, E.A. (2009) Menopausal symptoms following breast cancer treatment: A qualitative investigation of cognitive and behavioural responses. *Maturitas*, 63(4): 336–340.

Hunter, M.S., Gentry-Maharaj, A., Ryan, A., Burnell, M., Lanceley, A., Fraser, L. *et al.* (2012) Prevalence, frequency and problem-rating of hot flushes persist in older postmenopausal women: Impact of age, BMI, hysterectomy, lifestyle and mood in a cross-sectional cohort study of 10,418 British women aged 54–65. *British Journal of Obstetrics and Gynaecology*, 119: 40–50.

Hunter, M.S., Grunfeld, E.A., Mittal, S., Sikka, P., Ramirez, A.J. and Fentiman, I. (2004) Menopausal symptoms in women with breast cancer: Prevalence and treatment preferences. *Psycho-Oncology*, 13(11): 769–778.

Hunter, M.S., Gupta, P., Papitsch-Clark, A. and Sturdee, D.W. (2009c) Mid-aged health in women from the Indian subcontinent (MAH-WIS): A further quantitative and qualitative investigation of experience of menopause in UK Asian women, compared to UK Caucasian women and women living in Delhi. *Climacteric*, 12(1): 26–37.

Hunter, M.S. and Haqqani, J.R. (2011) An investigation of subjective perceptions and physiological measures of hot flushes and night sweats. *Climacteric*, 13(6): 146–151.

Hunter, M.S. and Liao, K.L.M. (1995) A psychological analysis of menopausal hot flushes. *British Journal of Clinical Psychology*, 34(4): 589–599.

Hunter, M.S. and Liao, K.L.M. (1996) Evaluation of a four-session cognitive-behavioural intervention for menopausal hot flushes. *British Journal of Health Psychology*, 1: 113–125.

Hunter, M.S. and Mann, E. (2010) A cognitive model of menopausal hot flushes. *Journal of Psychosomatic Research*, 69: 491–501.

Hunter, M.S. and O'Dea, I. (1997) Menopause: Bodily changes and multiple meanings. In Ussher, J.M. (Ed.) *Body Talk: The Material and Discursive Regulation of Sexuality, Madness and Reproduction*. London: Routledge, pp. 199–222.

Hunter, M.S. and O'Dea, I. (2001) Cognitive appraisal of the menopause: The menopause representations questionnaire (MRQ). *Psychology, Health & Medicine*, 6(1): 65–76.

Hunter, M.S., O'Dea, I. and Britten, N. (1997) Decision-making and hormone replacement therapy: A qualitative study. *Social Science Medicine*, 45(10): 1541–1548.

Hunter, M.S. and Rendall, M. (2007) Bio-psycho-socio-cultural perspectives on menopause. *Best Practice and Research Clinical Obstetrics & Gynaecology*, 21(2): 261–274.

Hunter, M.S. and Smith. M. (2015) *Managing hot flushes with cognitive behaviour therapy: a manual for health professionals*. London: Routledge.

Hunter, M.S. and Stefanopoulou, E. (2016) Vasomotor symptoms in prostate cancer survivors undergoing androgen deprivation therapy. *Climacteric*, 19: 91–97.

Hvas, L. (2006) Menopausal women's positive experience of growing older. *Maturitas*, 54: 245–251.

Judd, F.K., Hickey, M. and Bryant, C. (2012) Depression and midlife: Are we overpathologising the menopause? *Journal of Affective Disorders*, 136(3): 199–211.

Kabat-Zinn, J. (2003) Mindfulness-based interventions in context: Past, present, and future. *Clinical Psychology: Science and Practice*, 10(2): 144–156.

Kuh, D.L., Wadsworth, M. and Hardy, R. (1997) Women's health in midlife: The influence of the menopause, social factors and health in earlier life. *British Journal of Obstetrics and Gynaecology*, 104(8): 923–933.

Lang, I.A., Llewellyn, D.J., Hubbard, R.E., Langa, K.M. and Melzer, D. (2011) Income and the midlife peak in common mental disorder prevalence. *Psychological Medicine*, 41(7): 1365–1372.

Li, C., Samsioe, G., Borgfeldt, C., Lidfeldt, J., Agardh, C. and Nerbrand, C. (2003) Menopause related symptoms: What are the background factors? A prospective population-based cohort study of Swedish women. *American Journal of Obstetrics and Gynecology*, 189(6): 646–653.

Liao, L-M., Lunn, S. and Baker, M. (2014) Midlife menopause: Male partners talking. *Sexual Relationship Therapy*, 30(1): 167–180.

Maki, P.M., Kornstein, S.G., Joffe, H., Bromberger, J.T., Freeman, E.W., Athappilly, G. *et al.* (2019) Guidelines for the evaluation and treatment of perimenopausal depression: Summary and recommendations. *Journal of Women's Health*, 25(10): 1069–1085.

Mann, E., Smith, M.J., Balabanovic, J., Hellier, J., Hamed, H., Grunfeld, B. and Hunter, M.S. (2012) Efficacy of a cognitive behavioural intervention to treat menopausal symptoms following breast cancer treatment (MENOS 1): A randomized controlled trial. *Lancet Oncology*, 13: 309–318.

Manson, J.E., Hsia, J., Johnson, K.C., Rossouw, J.E., Assaf, A.R., Lasser, N.L. *et al.* (2003) Estrogen plus progestin and the risk of coronary heart disease. *New England Journal of Medicine*, 349: 523–534.

Marques, E.A., Mota, J. and Carvalho, J. (2012) Exercise effects on bone mineral density in older adults: A meta-analysis of randomized controlled trials. *Age*, 34(6): 1493–1515.

McCrone, P., Knapp, M., Kennedy, T., Darnley, S., Seed, P., Jones, R. *et al.* (2008) Cost-effectiveness of cognitive behaviour therapy in addition to mebeverine for irritable bowel syndrome. *European Journal of Gastrology and Hepatology*, 20: 255–263.

McKinlay, J.B., Travison, T.G., Araujo, A.B. and Kupelian, V. (2007) Male menopause: Time for a decent burial? *Menopause*, 14(6): 973–975.

Melby, M.K., Lock, M. and Kaufert, P. (2005) Culture and symptom reporting at menopause. *Human Reproductive Update*, 11: 495–512.

Menon, U., Burnell, M., Sharma, A., Gentry-Maharaj, A., Fraser, L., Parmar, M. *et al.* (2007) Decline in use of hormone therapy among postmenopausal women in the United Kingdom. *Menopause*, 14(3): 462–467.

Middleton, H., Shaw, I., Hull, S. and Feder, G. (2005) NICE guidelines for the management of depression. *British Medical Journal*, 330(7486): 267–268.

Mishra, G.D. and Kuh, D. (2012) Health symptoms during midlife in relation to menopausal transition: British prospective cohort study. *British Medical Journal*, 344: e402.

Mitchell, E.S. and Woods, N.F. (2011) Cognitive symptoms during the menopausal transition and early postmenopause. *Climacteric*, 14: 252–261.

Moorey, S., Greer, S. and Watson, M. (1994) Adjuvant psychological therapy for patients with cancer: Outcome at one year. *Psycho-Oncology*, 3: 39–46.

Morley, S., Eccleston, C. and Williams, A. (1999) Systematic review and meta-analysis of randomized controlled trials of cognitive behaviour therapy and behaviour therapy for chronic pain in adults, excluding headache. *Pain*, 80(1): 1–13.

National Institute for Health and Clinical Excellence (NICE). (2006) *Computerized Cognitive Behaviour Therapy for Depression and Anxiety: Technology Appraisal 97*. London: National Institute for Health and Clinical Excellence. Available at www. nice.org.uk.

National Institute for Health and Clinical Excellence (NICE). (2009) *Depression: The Treatment and Management of Depression in Adults (Update)*. Available at: www.nice.org.uk/guidance/CG90.

National Institute for Health and Care Excellence (NICE). (2015a) *NG28. Type 2 Diabetes in Adults: Management*. Available at www. nice.org.uk/guidance/ng28.

National Institutes of Health and Care Excellence (NICE). (2015b) *NICE Guidance on Diagnosis and Management of Menopause*. Available at: www.nice.org.uk/guidance/NG23.

NHS England. (2016) *Implementing the Five Year Forward View for Mental Health*. Available at www.england.nhs.uk/mentalhealth/taskforce/imp.

Nicolucci, A., Kovacs Burns, K., Holt, R.I., Comaschi, M., Hermanns, N., Ishii, H. *et al.* (2013) Diabetes attitudes, wishes and needs second study (DAWN2™): Cross-national benchmarking of diabetes-related psychosocial outcomes for people with diabetes. *Diabetic Medicine*, 30(7): 767–777.

North American Menopause Society (NAMS). (2015) Nonhormonal management of menopause-associated vasomotor symptoms: 2015 position statement of the North American menopause society. *Menopause*, 359: 1155–1172.

North American Menopause Society. (2010) Management of osteoporosis in postmenopausal women: 2010 position statement. *Menopause*, 17(1): 25–54.

Norton, S., Chilcot, J. and Hunter, M.S. (2014) Cognitive behaviour therapy for menopausal symptoms (hot flushes and night sweats):

Moderators and mediators of treatment effects. *Menopause*, 21: 574–578.

O'Dea, I., Hunter, M.S. and Anjos, S. (1999) Life satisfaction and health related quality of life (SF-36) of middle-aged men and women. *Climacteric*, 2: 131–140.

Office for National Statistics. (2010) *Cancer statistics registration: registration of cancer diagnosed in 2008*. London: Office for National Statistics.

Office for National Statistics. (2013) *Labour Market Statistics*. London: Office for National Statistics.

Otte, C. (2011) Cognitive behavioural therapy in anxiety disorders: Current state of the evidence. *Dialogues in Clinical Neuroscience*, 13(4): 413–421.

Padesky, C.A. and Mooney, K.A. (1990) Clinical tip: Presenting the cognitive model to patients. *International Cognitive Therapy Newsletter*, 6: 13–14.

Pampallona, S., Bollini, P., Tibaldi, G., Kupelnick, B. and Munizza, C. (2004) Combined pharmacotherapy and psychological treatment for depression: A systematic review. *Archives of General Psychiatry*, 61(7): 714–719.

Panay, N. and Fenton, A. (2008) Premature ovarian failure: A growing concern. *Climacteric*, 11: 1–3.

Parry, B.L. (2017) Beneficial effects of aging on mood in healthy postmenopausal women. *Menopause*, 24(5): 475–477.

Parton, C., Ussher, J.M. and Perz, J. (2017) Experiencing menopause in the context of cancer: Women's constructions of gendered subjectivities. *Psychology and Health*, 32(9): 1109–1126.

Paykel, E.S., Scott, J., Cornwall, P.L., Abbott, R., Crane, C., Pope, M. *et al.* (2005) Duration of relapse prevention after cognitive therapy in residual depression: Follow-up of controlled trial. *Psychological Medicine*, 35(1): 59–68.

Perz, J. and Ussher, J.M. (2008) 'The horror of this living decay': Women's negotiation and resistance of medical discourses around menopause and midlife. *Women's Studies International Forum*, 31: 293–299.

Pitkin, J. (2012) Alternative and complementary therapies for the menopause. *Menopause International*, 18: 20–27.

Prochaska, J.O. and Velicer, W.F. (1997) The transtheoretical model of health behaviour change. *American Journal of Health Promotion*, 12(1): 38–48.

Rashidi, A. and Shanley, D. (2009) Evolution of the menopause: Life histories and mechanisms. *Menopause International*, 15: 26–30.

Rendall, M.J., Simonds, L.M. and Hunter, M.S. (2008) The hot flush beliefs scale: A tool for assessing thoughts and beliefs associated with the experience of menopausal hot flushes and night sweats. *Maturitas*, 60(2): 158–169.

Reynolds, F. (1999) Some relationships between perceived control and women's reported coping strategies for menopausal hot flushes. *Maturitas*, 32: 25–32.

Reynolds, F. (2000) Relationships between catastrophic thoughts, perceived control and distress during menopausal hot flushes: Exploring the correlates of a questionnaire measure. *Maturitas*, 36: 113–122.

Rimer, J., Dwan, K., Lawlor, D.A., Greig, C.A., McMurdo, M., Morley, W. *et al.* (2012) Exercise for depression. *Cochrane Database Systematic Reviews*, 7: CD004366.

Rossouw, J.E., Anderson, G.L., Prentice, R.L., LaCroix, A.Z., Kooperberg, C., Stefanick, M.L. *et al.* (2002) Risks and benefits of oestrogen plus progestin in healthy postmenopausal women: Principal results from the women's health initiative randomized controlled trial. *Journal of the American Medical Association*, 288: 321–333.

Rubinstein, H.R. and Foster, J.L.H. (2013) 'I don't know whether it is to do with age or to do with hormones and whether it is do with a stage in your life': Making sense of menopause and the body. *Journal of Health Psychology*, 18: 292–307.

Sage, N., Sowden, M., Chorlton, E. and Edeleanu, A. (2008) *CBT for chronic illness and palliative care: a workbook and toolkit*. Chichester: John Wiley and Sons Ltd.

de Salis, I., Owen-Smith, A., Donovan, J.L. and Lawlor, D.A. (2018) Experiencing menopause in the UK: The interrelated narratives of normality, distress, and transformation. *Journal of Women & Aging*, 30(6): 520–540.

Salkovskis, P.M. (1991) The importance of behaviour in the maintenance of anxiety and panic: A cognitive account. *Behavioural Psychotherapy*, 19: 6–19.

Sassarini, J., Perera, M., Spowart, K., McAllister, K., Judith Fraser, Glasspool, R., et al. (2018) Managing vulvovaginal atrophy after breast cancer. *Post Reproductive Health*, 24(4): 163–165.

Sayakhot, P., Vincent, A. and Teede, H. (2012) Cross-cultural study: Experience, understanding of menopause, and related therapies in Australian and Laotian women. *Menopause*, 19(12): 1300–1308.

Sergeant, J. and Rizq, R. (2017) 'It's all part of the big "change"': A grounded theory study of women's identity during menopause. *Journal of Psychosomatic Obstetrics & Gynecology*, 38: 189–201.

Showalter, E. (1987) *The female malady*. London: Virago.

Sievert, L.L., Obermayer, C.M. and Price, K. (2006) Determinants of hot flashes and night sweats. *Annals of Human Biology*, 33: 4–16.

Singer, D., Mann, E., Hunter, M.S., Pitkin, J. and Panay, N. (2011) The silent grief: Psychosocial aspects of premature ovarian failure. *Climacteric*, 14(4): 428–437.

Singh-Manoux, A., Kivimaki, M., Glymour, M.M., Elbaz, A., Berr, C., Ebmeier, K.P. *et al.* (2012) Timing of onset of cognitive decline: Results from Whitehall II prospective cohort study. *British Medical Journal*, 344: d7622.

Slade, P. and Amaee, S. (1995) The role of anxiety and temperature in the experience of menopausal hot flushes. *Journal of Reproductive and Infant Psychology*, 13(2): 127–133.

Smith, M.J., Mann, E., Mirza, A. and Hunter, M.S. (2011) Men and women's perceptions of hot flushes within social situations: Are menopausal women's negative beliefs valid? *Maturitas*, 69: 57–62.

Sprague, B.L., Trentham-Dietz, A. and Cronin, K.A.A. (2012) Sustained decline in postmenopausal hormone use: Results from the national health and nutrition examination survey, 1999–2010. *Obstetrics & Gynecology*, 120(3): 595–603.

Stefanopoulou, E., Yousaf, O., Grunfeld, E.A. and Hunter, M.S. (2015) A randomised controlled trial of a brief cognitive behavioural intervention for men who have hot flushes following prostate cancer treatment (MANCAN). *Psycho-Oncology*, 24(9): 1159–1166.

Swartzman, L.C., Edelberg, R. and Kemmann, E. (1990) Impact of stress on objectively recorded menopausal hot flushes and on flush report bias. *Health Psychology*, 9(5): 529–545.

Taylor, R.R. (2005) The psychological complexities of chronic illness and impairment. In Taylor, R.R. (Ed.) *Cognitive Behavioral Therapy for Chronic Illness and Disability*. New York: Springer, pp. 22–23.

Teasdale, J.D., Segal, Z.V., Williams, J.M.G., Ridgeway, V.A., Soulsby, J.M. and Lau, M.A. (2000) Prevention of relapse/recurrence in major depression by mindfulness-based cognitive therapy. *Journal of Consulting and Clinical Psychology*, 68: 615–623.

Thurston, R.C., Sowers, M.F.R., Sternfeld, B., Gold, E.B., Bromberger, J., Chang, Y. *et al.* (2009) Gains in body fat and vasomotor symptom reporting over the menopausal transition. The study of women's health across the nation (SWAN). *American Journal of Epidemiology*, 170(6): 766–774.

Thurston, R.C., Sowers, M.F.R., Sutton-Tyrrell, K., Everson-Rose, S.A., Lewis, T.T., Edmundowicz, D. *et al.* (2008) Abdominal adiposity and hot flashes among midlife women. *Menopause*, 15: 429–434.

Tworoger, S.S., Chubak, J., Aiello, E.J., Yasui, Y., Ulrich, C.M., Farin, F.M. *et al.* (2004) The effect of *CYP19* and *COMT* polymorphisms on exercise-induced fat loss in postmenopausal women. *Obesity Research*, 12: 72–981.

Ussher, J.M., Perz, J., Gilbert, E., Wong, W.K.T. and Hobbs, K. (2013) Renegotiating sex and intimacy after cancer: Resisting the coital imperative. *Cancer Nursing*, 36(6): 454–462.

Utian, W.H. (2008) Memory, menopause and hormones: Conclusions from the North American menopause society 2008 hormone therapy position statement. *Menopause Management*, September–October: 6–7.

Verheul, H.A.M., Coelingh-Bennink, H.J.T., Kenemans, P., Atsma, W.J., Burger, C.W., Eden, J.A. *et al.* (2000) Effects of estrogens and hormone replacement therapy on breast cancer risk and on efficacy of breast cancer therapies. *Maturitas*, 36(1): 1–17.

Vivian-Taylor, J. and Hickey, M. (2014) Menopause and depression: Is there a link? *Maturitas*, 79(2): 142–146.

Warwick, H. and Salkovskis, P.M. (1990) Hypochondriasis. *Behaviour Research and Therapy*, 28(2): 105–117.

White, C.A. (2001) *Cognitive behaviour therapy for chronic medical problems: a guide to assessment and treatment in practice*. Chichester: John Wiley & Sons Ltd.

Whitfield, G. and Williams, C. (2003) The evidence base for cognitive-behavioural therapy in depression: Delivery in busy clinical settings. *Advances in Psychiatric Treatment*, 9(1): 21–30.

Wilbush, J. (1979) La Menespausie – the birth of a syndrome. *Maturitas*, 1: 145–151.

Wilson, R.A. (1966) *Feminine Forever*. New York: Evans, p. 43.

Winterich, J.A. (2003) Sex, menopause and culture: Sexual orientation and the meaning of menopause for women's sex lives. *Gender and Society*, 17(4): 627–642.

Woods, N.F., Mariella, A. and Mitchell, E.S. (2006) Depressed mood symptoms during the menopausal transition: Observations from the Seattle midlife women's health study. *Climacteric*, 9: 195–203.

Woods, N.F. and Mitchell, E.S. (2010) Sleep symptoms during the menopausal transition and early postmenopause: Observations from the Seattle midlife women's health study. *Sleep*, 33: 539–549.

Woods, N.F., Mitchell, E.S. and Landis, C. (2005) Anxiety, hormonal changes, and vasomotor symptoms during the menopause transition. *Menopause*, 12(3): 242–245.

Woyka, J. (2017) Consensus statement for non-hormonal-based treatments for menopausal symptoms. *Post Reproductive Health*, 23(2): 71–75.

Ziv-Gal, A. and Flaws, J.A. (2010) Factors that may influence the experience of hot flushes by healthy middle-aged women. *Journal of Women's Health*, 19(10): 1905–1914.

Index

Page numbers in italic indicate a figure and page numbers in bold indicate a table on the corresponding page.

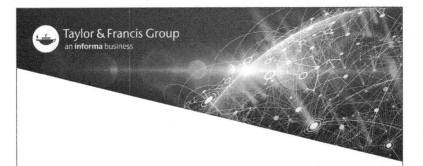